NAVIGATING THE FERTILITY MAZE

TAKE CHARGE OF YOUR REPRODUCTIVE HEALTH
AND ACHIEVE YOUR DREAM OF PARENTHOOD

KASIA MARSHALL

© **Copyright 2023 - All rights reserved.**

The content contained within this book may not be reproduced, duplicated, or transmitted without direct written permission from the author or the publisher.

Under no circumstances will any blame or legal responsibility be held against the publisher, or author, for any damages, reparation, or monetary loss due to the information contained within this book, either directly or indirectly.

Legal Notice:

This book is copyright protected. It is only for personal use. You cannot amend, distribute, sell, use, quote or paraphrase any part, or the content within this book, without the consent of the author or publisher.

Disclaimer Notice:

Please note the information contained within this document is for educational and entertainment purposes only. All effort has been executed to present accurate, up to date, reliable, complete information. No warranties of any kind are declared or implied. Readers acknowledge that the author is not engaged in the rendering of legal, financial, medical or professional advice. The content within this book has been derived from various sources. Please consult a licensed professional before attempting any techniques outlined in this book.

By reading this document, the reader agrees that under no circumstances is the author responsible for any losses, direct or indirect, that are incurred as a result of the use of the information contained within this document, including, but not limited to, errors, omissions, or inaccuracies.

CONTENTS

Introduction ... 7

1. FERTILE GROUNDS—UNRAVELING THE MYSTERIES OF FERTILITY ... 13
   Defining Infertility ... 13
   Breaking Stereotypes: It's Not Just Her Problem ... 15
   When to Seek Help ... 17
   The Path to Treatment: Hope Renewed ... 17
   Success Stories: Understanding the Odds ... 19

2. THE MENSTRUAL CYCLE—A KEY TO FERTILITY ... 25
   Menstrual Cycle Overview ... 26
   Five Myths About Female Fertility ... 31
   The Role of Hormones in Fertility ... 33

3. CONCEIVING DREAMS—PREPARING FOR PREGNANCY ... 37
   Setting Goals ... 39
   Diet ... 43
   Exercise ... 49
   Weight ... 53

4. EMBARKING ON PARENTHOOD—CONCEPTION OPTIMIZATION ... 57
   The Best Times for Conception ... 59
   Tracking Ovulation and Fertility Signs ... 61
   Strategies for Enhancing Fertility During Intercourse ... 65

5. SILENT STRUGGLES—FEMALE
   INFERTILITY   71
   The Dance of Conception: A Precise
   Choreography   73
   The Causes of Female Infertility   74
   Diagnosing and Assessing Fertility Issues   77

6. SCIENCE AND HOPE UNITE—
   EXPLORING ART   83
   Davina and Barry: Triumph Over Infertility   83
   IVF   85
   Intrauterine Insemination (IUI)   101
   The Emotional Journey of Fertility
   Treatments   109

7. WHISPERS OF STRENGTH—HEALING
   AND HOPE AFTER PREGNANCY LOSS   117
   Laura and Bex's Paths Intersect   117
   Miscarriages and Pregnancy Loss   120
   Emotional Healing and Support After Loss   130

8. BLOSSOM   143
   Aleiya and Michal's Story   143
   The Importance of a Healthy Lifestyle   146
   Obesity and Eating Disorders: A Weighty
   Matter for Fertility   149
   Nutritional Altitude and Sperm Quality   151
   Physical Exercise: Balancing Act   153
   The Invisible Culprits: Anxiety, Depression,
   and Misconception   155
   Destressing When You're Trying to
   Conceive   161

9. THE BEGINNING—THE FIRST
   TRIMESTER EXPERIENCE   167
   Emma's Miracle: Our Journey of Hope   167
   Early Pregnancy Symptoms and Changes   169
   Pregnancy Myths: Debunking the Bumps   172
   Your First Doctor's Appointment   175

Conclusion	181
Glossary	185
References	189

INTRODUCTION

> *A baby is something you carry inside you for nine months, in your arms for three years, and in your heart until the day you die.*
>
> — MARY MASON

Every weekend, it seemed like another friend was celebrating the imminent arrival of a new life. Baby showers and gender reveal parties had become a regular part of our social calendar, painting a vivid picture of the vibrant tapestry of parenthood that surrounded us. Yet, as my partner and I navigated the ebbs and flows of these joyous occasions, we found ourselves on a parallel journey —one marked by its unique challenges and uncertainties. During these occasions, a famous quote would dance before my mind's eye, filling me with tears I could not shed until I could reach the sanctuary of our home, whose silence was fast becoming a constant reminder in and of itself.

Sitting among the laughter, balloons, and pastel-colored onesies, I couldn't help but wonder if our story would someday intersect with those of our friends, with the joyful echoes of children's laughter and playdates filling that deafening silence of our home.

But as the weeks turned into months, and then years, and all our friends were starting to bond with other friends with kids around the same age, which automatically left us out, not only did our circle grow smaller, but so did our hopes start to diminish. The journey toward parenthood that seemed so exciting to others had become an uphill climb for us, marked by dashed hopes and silent prayers. The seemingly simple act of conceiving a child became an intricate puzzle, whose pieces eluded our grasp.

Each of us embarks on the life's journey with unique dreams and aspirations, and for many like us, the dream of becoming a parent lies at the core of their heart's desires. But the path to parenthood is not always straightforward; it can be riddled with unexpected hurdles, turning dreams into tests of endurance and emotional resilience. The process of creating life is a symphony of intricacies, where every note must be in tune for the crescendo of conception to resound.

As a mother of two precious gifts, I can tell you that our going through the most for all those years was certainly worth every ounce of angst. Yes, our efforts were finally rewarded; however, I also know of friends we've made along the way who were unable to conceive, not for want of doing everything they possibly could to get there.

The fact that you are reading this book means that you are at one of the stages along the way. And while our road may be arduous with an uncertain ending, you will emerge a more resilient, stronger, and more compassionate person than you were at the start, irrespective of the outcome of your efforts. Please stick with me as we go through the gauntlet together.

Infertility is a term that carries more weight than its mere syllables. It encompasses the stories of countless individuals and couples, each grappling with the profound emotions of the struggle to conceive. It is a multifaceted challenge that defies simple explanations, affecting both women and men, weaving a complex narrative that intertwines biology, time, and fate. Defined as the inability to conceive after a year of unprotected intimacy, infertility casts a shadow over the lives of millions across the globe. In the United States, where the pursuit of happiness often includes the dream of parenthood, statistics reveal that approximately one in five married women aged 15 to 49, with no prior births, face the reality of infertility (Centers for Disease Control and Prevention, 2019). This statistic isn't just a number; it's a chorus of dreams deferred, a choir of heartache, and a reminder that life's journey doesn't always unfold as planned.

As age paints its brushstrokes upon the canvas of our lives, fertility becomes a complex tapestry where threads of possibility and limitation are woven together. While the journey is often more challenging for women, age is a shared factor that shapes the experience for both partners. With time, the story of fertility unfolds with ever-increasing urgency, a narrative that can't be ignored or put on hold.

However, for us, the road to parenthood is not without hope. Amid the challenges and uncertainties, there shines a guiding light in the form of reproductive endocrinologists—medical experts who specialize in navigating the labyrinthine complexities of fertility. Their expertise is a beacon of hope, a reminder that science, combined with empathy and personalized care, can illuminate the darkest corners of infertility.

In the pages that follow, we'll embark on a journey of understanding, peeling back the layers of fertility challenges that women like us face. From the intricacies of ovulation to the impact of age, we'll explore the factors that shape the path to conception. We'll shine a light on male infertility, dispelling the myth that the journey toward parenthood is solely a woman's burden.

As we navigate this sea of emotions and scientific knowledge, remember that you are not alone on this voyage.

Others have walked this path before, leaving behind stories of resilience, strength, and triumph. Armed with knowledge and supported by a dedicated medical team, the journey toward parenthood becomes a joint venture, one where the complexities of biology are met with the power of the human spirit.

In the chapters to come, we'll unveil the multifaceted dimensions of fertility challenges, delivering into disrupted ovulation patterns, fallopian tube obstructions, and the significance of the uterine environment. We'll embrace age as a guiding force, understanding its influence and role in shaping our narratives. Alongside the scientific exploration, we'll honor the personal stories of those who have embarked on this journey, their courage and determination inspiring us all.

Together, we'll step into the heart of fertility's uncharted waters, armed with the tools to understand, the knowledge to navigate, and the compass to offer solace. The journey may be challenging, but remember, it's also a testament to the remarkable resilience of the human spirit. The road to parenthood may be winding, but every step is a testimony to the beauty of hope, the strength of love, and the unwavering pursuit of a dream.

1

FERTILE GROUNDS—UNRAVELING THE MYSTERIES OF FERTILITY

"If you've dabbled in every trying to conceive (TTC) trick ever shared in those women's circles and still found yourself on the disappointing end, take heart! You're definitely not alone in this rollercoaster of a journey. And guess what? There's no magical one-size-fits-all solution."

— GUTTUSSO, 2011

DEFINING INFERTILITY

Infertility is basically when you've been trying to get pregnant, doing the baby dance, for a whole year (or longer) without any luck. Now, if you happen to be a bit wiser and wonderful, aged 35 or older, some doctors might start checking things out after just six months of unprotected romance (Centers for Disease Control and Prevention, 2019). But remember, these definitions are primarily for keeping tabs on things, not for telling you what to do.

Let me hit you with a few stats from which you will see hope and challenges thrown into the mix.

The Statistics of Hope and Challenge

In the United States, approximately 19% of married women between the ages of 15 and 49 who have not previously given birth experience infertility, defined as the inability to conceive after one year of trying. Moreover, within this same demographic, around 26% of women face challenges in either conceiving or maintaining a pregnancy to full term, a condition referred to as impaired fecundity, as reported by the Centers for Disease Control and Prevention (2019).

The prevalence of infertility and impaired fecundity is notably lower among married women aged 15 to 49 years who have given birth at least once. In this category, approximately six percent experience infertility, which signifies the inability to conceive after one year of trying, while 14% encounter challenges in conceiving or sustaining a pregnancy to full term (Centers for Disease Control and Prevention, 2019).

BREAKING STEREOTYPES: IT'S NOT JUST HER PROBLEM

Infertility is not always a woman's problem. Both men and women can contribute to infertility. Infertility in men can be caused by different factors and is typically evaluated by a semen analysis (Centers for Disease Control and Prevention, 2019). During a semen analysis, a specialized assessment is conducted to assess parameters such as sperm concentration, motility (sperm movement), and morphology (sperm shape). It is important to note that semen analysis showing slight abnormalities does not automatically indicate male infertility. Instead, the purpose of a semen analysis is to assist in identifying the extent to which male factors may play a role in infertility.

Disruption of testicular or ejaculatory function, varicocele, trauma to the testes, heavy alcohol use, smoking, anabolic steroid use, cancer treatment, medical conditions, hormonal disorders, and genetic disorders are all potential contributors to male infertility (Centers for Disease Control and Prevention, 2019).

While advanced age predominantly serves as a significant factor in predicting female infertility, couples in which the male partner is 40 years or older tend to be more prone to encountering challenges when attempting to conceive. Being overweight or obese, smoking, excessive alcohol and drug use, exposure to testosterone, radiation, high testicular temperatures, certain medications, and environmental toxins can also influence male fertility (Centers for Disease Control and Prevention, 2019).

Female Fertility—a Race Against Time

Women need several vital reproductive organs to conceive. Conditions affecting any one of these organs can contribute to female infertility. Some of these conditions include disruption of ovarian function, fallopian tube obstruction, and physical characteristics of the uterus.

The Waning Influence of Age

Female fertility is known to decline with age. Roughly 22% of married couples with women aged 30 to 39 face challenges when attempting to conceive their first child, in contrast to approximately 13% of married couples where the woman is under 30. The decline in fertility with increasing age can be attributed to the deterioration of egg quality over time. Additionally, older women tend to have a diminished ovarian reserve, and they are at a higher risk of experiencing health conditions that can contribute to fertility issues. Aging also increases a woman's chances of miscarriage and of having a child with a genetic abnormality (Centers for Disease Control and Prevention, 2019).

WHEN TO SEEK HELP

A woman's chances of having a baby decrease rapidly every year after age 30. The general consensus among experts is that women under 35 who do not have evident health or fertility issues and maintain regular menstrual cycles should aim to conceive for a minimum of one year before seeking medical advice. However, for women aged 35 years or older, couples should see a healthcare provider after six months of trying unsuccessfully. Women over the age of 40 years may consider seeking more immediate evaluation and treatment.

Some health problems also increase the risk of infertility. So, couples with certain signs or symptoms should not delay seeing their healthcare provider when trying to fall pregnant. Indicators or manifestations encompass irregular or absent menstrual cycles, a history of pelvic inflammatory disease, endometriosis, known or suspected uterine or tubal conditions, a history of multiple miscarriages, and genetic or acquired factors that increase the likelihood of diminished ovarian reserve (Centers for Disease Control and Prevention, 2019).

THE PATH TO TREATMENT: HOPE RENEWED

Doctors will begin by collecting medical and sexual history from both partners. The initial evaluation usually includes a semen analysis, a tubal evaluation, and ovarian reserve testing. The good news is that there is hope.

Infertility can be treated with medicine, surgery, intrauterine insemination, or assisted reproductive technology. The treatment choice depends on various factors, including the cause of infertility, its duration, the female partner's age, and personal preferences.

Harnessing the Power of Medicine

Some common medicines used to treat infertility in women include clomiphene citrate, letrozole, human menopausal gonadotropin (hMG), follicle-stimulating hormone (FSH), gonadotropin-releasing hormone (GnRH) analogs, GnRH antagonists, metformin, bromocriptine, and cabergoline (Centers for Disease Control and Prevention, 2019).

Intrauterine insemination (IUI) is a commonly referred to infertility treatment known as artificial insemination. This procedure involves the introduction of specially processed sperm into the woman's uterus. On occasion, prior to IUI, the woman may also receive medication to stimulate ovulation.

Assisted reproductive technology (ART) encompasses all fertility interventions where either eggs or embryos are manipulated externally. The primary type of ART is in vitro fertilization (IVF), which involves removing mature eggs from a woman's ovaries, combining them with sperm in the laboratory, and returning the embryos to the woman's body or donating them to another woman (Centers for Disease Control and Prevention, 2019).

SUCCESS STORIES: UNDERSTANDING THE ODDS

The probability of success in assisted reproductive technology (ART) treatments can fluctuate significantly, contingent upon various elements such as the clinic performing the procedure, the infertility diagnosis, and the age of the woman undergoing the procedure. This last factor—the woman's age—is especially important.

While ART procedures can be financially burdensome and require a substantial investment of time, they have proven to be a valuable means by which numerous couples have realized their dreams of parenthood. The most common complication of ART is multiple pregnancies, which can be prevented or minimized by limiting the number of embryos transferred (Centers for Disease Control and Prevention, 2019).

IVF, intracytoplasmic sperm injection (ICSI), zygote intrafallopian transfer (ZIFT), and gamete intrafallopian transfer (GIFT) are some of the ART methods, each with its unique approach to overcoming infertility (Centers for Disease Control and Prevention, 2019).

Imagine spending most of our young adult years trying not to get pregnant until we're ready to start a family, that is. Then, we struggle to conceive. According to the CDC, estimates place the number of couples who struggle with fertility in the United States alone is more than 10% or roughly one in ten (Guttusso, 2011). I want you to take heart, be patient, and relax because there is hope yet—like these couples discovered:

The Hixons

The Hixons started trying to conceive in February 2012, even though Tia had also tried for several years before that with her first partner. At first, doctors were baffled, and it was only in 2014 that it was discovered that Tia had polycystic ovary syndrome (PCOS). As you may know, this means that Tia's estrogen levels were too high, limiting her ability to conceive (Guttusso, 2011).

Of course, like most of us, the Hixons tried every method they learned about, from the conventional ones to performing acrobatics in the bedroom—nothing worked. Then, their doctor prescribed an ovulation stimulator called Clomid. This treatment worked incredibly fast. "I took my first round of five pills on May 7 and had my first positive pregnancy test on June 8," beamed Tia tearfully (Guttusso, 2011).

When asked what advice they would give to other couples struggling to fall pregnant, this is what they said:

"Play with each other. This part of your journey is the most trying experience. Especially since you suddenly become acutely aware of all the pregnant couples, children, baby products, and happy families around you. It can be utterly overwhelming. But, as hard as it can be, try to focus on the gift you already have: a loving partner who is on this journey with you. Share your pain, supporting and encouraging each other to never give up. Confide in those you trust. Trying unsuccessfully to conceive can feel like you're grieving for your child you haven't met yet. Feel what you feel. Never stop believing in the impossible. Brace for those hormonal changes. Most of all, be kind to yourself and each other on this frustrating journey to conception" (Guttusso, 2011).

Celebrity Couples

No one is immune to fertility challenges, including celebrities. Some have been more public about their struggles over the years, while others have remained more private about it.

Emma Thompson and Greg Wise

Although this delightful couple have two children, they have been open about their fertility journey and admit that their daughter Gaia was conceived through IVF. Greg said IVF was horrible. "You're filling your partner full of drugs all the time. Your fertility cuts to the root of yourself as a being, especially as a woman. You have the potential of producing life and if there's a glitch...I think even now there are still a lot who think that you're not a whole woman" (Kirkwin-Jones, 2023).

Hugh Jackman and Deborra-Lee Furness

The journey to parenthood had been long, difficult, and intensely sorrowful. Hugh opened up about this part of their private lives:

"We didn't know where in the process that would happen but biologically obviously we tried, and it was not happening for us, and it is a difficult time. We did IVF, and Deb had a couple of miscarriages. I'll never forget it—the miscarriage thing—it happens to one in three pregnancies, but it's very, very rarely talked about" (Kirkwin-Jones, 2023).

The celebrity couple of over 26 years have opted to adopt. They have two children, Oscar and Ava. Oscar, now 22, was adopted in 2000, while their daughter, Ava, now 18, was adopted in 2005 (Weiss, 2023).

The list of couples, celebrity or otherwise, who are struggling with fertility is more extensive than you might think. Fortunately, there are loads of options available to us these days. Donor eggs, donor sperm, donated embryos, and gestational carriers are options for those facing complex fertility challenges or genetic issues. These options redefine the boundaries of parenthood, offering hope to those who might otherwise have none (Centers for Disease Control and Prevention, 2019).

If you want to go into the more cutting-edge developments in fertility treatments, preimplantation genetic testing (PGT) is a procedure used to identify genetic disorders or chromosomal abnormalities in embryos created during an IVF cycle. This process helps ensure healthy pregnancies and births, particularly for those at risk of passing on genetic conditions (Centers for Disease Control and Prevention, 2019).

If you've been trying to conceive for a while and have started to wonder if it might be time to consult the experts, I hope you've found the answer in this chapter and are somewhat more relaxed about the next steps. Now that you know just how many options there are out there and have read the miraculous success stories so far (there are more to come), you should feel more confident and reassured about your journey toward pregnancy and your fertility.

Of course, the key to unlocking the magic of conception lies in that musical moon cycle of menstruation. In the following chapter, we will explore the all-important menstrual cycle, a few myths and truths about conception, age, and the role of hormones.

2

THE MENSTRUAL CYCLE—A KEY TO FERTILITY

"Everything is very number fixated, your egg count, hormone level, sperm count—even my age was a big issue. It just consumed me. To the average person, I looked young at that time, but inside I felt hollow, that my body was failing me and that I was a failure, a failure in general. How can this not work, if you try hard enough, things should happen, but it just wasn't.

I describe the trying period as one of the darker times of my life and it was only long after that I could even talk about it. I believe that the baby would come to you if you are receptive, whether it's adoption, IVF, or naturally. What I would tell anyone is that when you get that positive test, when your baby comes, all that emotion, pain and angst goes away—because then it doesn't matter."

— MOLLY, U.S.A. (CLEARBLUE, 2021).

Like Molly, thousands, if not millions of women, discover on the painful journey to parenthood that we are at the mercy of our body's chemistry and menstrual cycle.

The menstrual cycle, a marvel of our biology, is a rhythmic and intricate dance orchestrated by hormones, and it plays a fundamental role in a person's fertility. It's a process that unfolds in four distinct phases: menstruation, follicular, ovulation, and luteal. In this section, we will delve into the depths of this crucial piece in the fertility puzzle by examining its significance, key milestones, phases, and common issues while emphasizing the importance of seeking medical assistance when needed (*Menstrual Cycle*, 2012).

MENSTRUAL CYCLE OVERVIEW

At its core, the menstrual cycle is a symphony directed by hormones, resulting in the regular shedding of the uterine lining, commonly known as "periods." This cyclic phenomenon resembles a monthly reset button for the female body. It's a process that starts anew with each period, preparing the body for the potential miracle of life (*Menstrual Cycle*, 2012). Estrogen and progesterone are the primary hormones that regulate the menstrual cycle. These hormones guide the uterine lining's growth and subsequent shedding *Menstrual Cycle*, 2012). This shedding is what most people experience as their monthly period.

Understanding the Menstrual Cycle

A profound understanding of the menstrual cycle reveals its awe-inspiring purpose: preparing the female body for pregnancy. If conception doesn't occur, the body efficiently disposes of the nurturing environment it has created. Think of it as an artist who prepares a canvas for a masterpiece, but if the masterpiece isn't completed, the canvas is gently wiped clean to start afresh, each month offering a new opportunity for creation (*Menstrual Cycle*, 2012).

Tracking and Cycle Duration

The menstrual cycle is as unique as the individual experiencing it. Tracking involves measuring the time from the first day of one period to the first day of the next. While an average cycle spans 28–29 days, it's essential to acknowledge that this average masks considerable variability. Some people have shorter cycles, lasting around 21 days, while others have longer ones, extending up to 35 days or even more. These variations are entirely normal and are part of the rich tapestry of human biology (*Menstrual Cycle*, 2012).

Key Milestones: Menarche and Menopause

Two significant milestones punctuate a person's reproductive journey. The first period, known as menarche, usually occurs around the age of 12–13, although it can vary (*Menstrual Cycle*, 2012). On the other end of the spectrum, we have menopause, which marks the end of the reproductive years, with an average age of 51–52. However, this can happen later or earlier for some individuals. These milestones are unique, and each person's journey is her own (*Menstrual Cycle*, 2012).

Phases of the Menstrual Cycle

Understanding the phases of the menstrual cycle can provide insights into fertility and reproductive health (*Menstrual Cycle*, 2012):

Phase 1: Menstruation

This is the beginning of the cycle and a time when the body sheds the uterine lining, which has been prepared for pregnancy. Menstruation typically lasts for three to seven days and is often accompanied by varying levels of discomfort or pain.

Phase 2: Follicular Phase

Starting on the first day of menstruation, this phase spans approximately 13–14 days. The uterine lining thickens during this time in anticipation of potential embryo implantation. Hormones like follicle-stimulating hormone (FSH) and luteinizing hormone (LH) play critical roles in this phase.

Phase 3: Ovulation

Ovulation is a pivotal moment that occurs approximately midway through the menstrual cycle, typically around day 14 in a 28-day cycle. An egg is released from the ovary, marking the fertile window, which usually spans 16–32 hours. It's a brief but crucial period for conception.

Phase 4: Luteal Phase

The luteal phase begins after ovulation, lasting around 12–14 days. During this phase, the uterine lining continues to thicken, and the corpus luteum, a temporary endocrine gland formed from the ruptured ovarian follicle, produces progesterone, which is crucial for maintaining early pregnancy.

Common Menstrual Problems

While the menstrual cycle is a vital aspect of reproductive health, for a large number of women, it is not without its challenges (*Menstrual Cycle*, 2012):

- **PMS (Premenstrual Syndrome):** Many individuals experience emotional and physical symptoms in the days leading up to menstruation.

These symptoms can include mood swings, bloating, and breast tenderness.
- **Dysmenorrhea (Painful Periods):** Painful menstrual cramps can be debilitating for some. They can result from the uterine muscles contracting to expel the uterine lining.
- **Heavy Bleeding:** Some people experience heavy menstrual bleeding (menorrhagia), which can lead to fatigue and discomfort.
- **Amenorrhea (Absence of Periods):** The absence of periods can occur due to various reasons, including stress, intense physical training, or underlying medical conditions.

Seeking Medical Help

Your menstrual cycle is a reflection of your overall health. Any significant changes in your cycle patterns, such as heavy bleeding, excessively long or short cycles, persistent pain, or irregularities that deviate significantly from your usual experience, should prompt a conversation with a healthcare provider. Their expertise can provide valuable insights, offer relief from discomfort, and address any underlying health concerns you may have (*Menstrual Cycle*, 2012).

FIVE MYTHS ABOUT FEMALE FERTILITY

When it comes to fertility and the journey to parenthood, misconceptions abound. Well-meaning friends and family often share advice, but it's essential to separate fact from fiction, especially when your fertility and potential family are at stake. Let's dispel five common myths (Kutteh et al., n.d.):

Myth 1: Few Women Suffer From Infertility—Most Women Get Pregnant Easily

In the United States, about 15% of couples encounter fertility challenges, with many receiving a diagnosis of a reproductive disorder. If you're under 35, experts suggest trying to conceive for about a year before seeking medical assistance. However, if you have noticeable issues like irregular periods or known pelvic adhesions, don't wait a year. For women aged 35 and older, consulting a doctor is advisable after six months of trying without success.

Myth 2: Infertility Is Solely a Woman's Issue

You will be astounded to note that in approximately 50% of couples facing infertility, male factors or sperm disorders are the culprits. These issues can involve sperm count, sperm shape, or their ability to move effectively. Notably, many men with low or no sperm production have treatable conditions, underscoring the need for early testing during infertility evaluations.

Myth 3: Age Does Not Affect Fertility if You're Healthy

The impact of age on fertility is undeniable. Fertility treatments, including IVF, can help, but a woman's chances of getting pregnant decrease as she gets older. By age 35, the likelihood of conception is about half what it was between the ages of 19 and 26. After 38, both egg quantity and quality decline significantly. Seeking help early can make a substantial difference in achieving pregnancy.

Myth 4: Conception Is Easy After Having One Child

Secondary fertility challenges, affecting couples who already have one child but struggle to conceive again, are more common than one might think, affecting over 3 million people in the U.S. alone. These issues often stem from the same factors as primary fertility problems, such as pelvic scarring, endometriosis, blocked fallopian tubes, or age-related factors. Treatments for primary and secondary fertility issues are generally the same.

Myth 5: Stress Causes Infertility. Relax and You'll Get Pregnant

While stress can affect ovulation under extreme circumstances, it's not a direct cause of infertility for most couples. While stress-reduction practices like yoga and acupuncture can positively affect overall well-being, they haven't been proven to offer a definitive fertility benefit.

So, don't let myths deter you from your path to parenthood. Fertility challenges are common and can affect anyone. If you've been trying to conceive for an extended period without success, contact a specialist. They have the expertise and resources to help guide you on your journey to building your family, offering hope and solutions to those navigating the complex landscape of fertility.

THE ROLE OF HORMONES IN FERTILITY

Fertility, the miracle of human reproduction, is an intricate journey guided by a symphony of hormones. These natural fluctuations in hormone levels orchestrate the complex dance of the menstrual cycle, playing a pivotal role in a woman's ability to conceive and carry a pregnancy to term. In exploring the role of hormones in fertility, we unravel the intricate web of four key female fertility hormones: FSH, LH, oestradiol (estradiol or estrogen), and progesterone (*What Are the Key Fertility Hormones*, 2020).

The Menstrual Cycle: A Ballet of Hormones

A woman's menstrual cycle is a unique and delicate process, encompassing various phases that prepare the body for potential pregnancy. Understanding the interplay of hormones during this cycle is crucial for those planning to start a family (*What Are the Key Fertility Hormones*, 2020).

Follicular Phase: FSH and Oestradiol

The journey begins with the follicular phase, starting on the first day of the menstrual cycle. During this stage, FSH takes center stage, stimulating the growth of ovarian follicles in preparation for ovulation. At the same time, oestradiol, which is a type of estrogen produced by the ovaries, starts to rise. Oestradiol facilitates the development of the egg within the follicle, preparing for its release.

Luteal Phase: Progesterone's Reign

After an egg is released from the ovary, the luteal phase takes over, lasting for approximately 14 days. Progesterone steps into the spotlight during this phase, produced by the corpus luteum—a structure formed when the follicle ruptures and releases its egg. Progesterone plays a vital role in preparing the uterine lining for the potential implantation of that much anticipated fertilized egg. If pregnancy does not occur, progesterone levels start to wane, and the menstrual cycle reboots.

LH: Orchestrating Ovulation

LH, another crucial player, is produced by the pituitary gland in the brain. LH is responsible for regulating the function of the ovaries in women. It is LH that triggers the release of an egg from the ovary. This process is known as ovulation—recognized as the pivotal event that offers a sliver of opportunity for conception to take place.

You'd best hurry, though; this window of opportunity is short-lived.

Age and Fertility: A Delicate Balance

We cannot discuss fertility hormones without considering age. Female fertility peaks during the early twenties but starts to decline in the mid-thirties. As age advances, the quantity and quality of eggs diminish, making conception more challenging.

Living in the hope that your chemistry and hormones achieve that magic balance can become your principal obsession at this point, but that's okay. It is a great place to start when embarking on the serious stages of trying to conceive. In the next chapter, we get down to the serious business of setting goals and consulting your doctor about the best ways to prepare your body for pregnancy by making healthy lifestyle choices—the dos and don'ts of this crucial preparation stage. Diet and exercise are more critical to conception than you may think. A healthy lifestyle combined with a winning attitude are sure to escalate your chances of conception.

3

CONCEIVING DREAMS— PREPARING FOR PREGNANCY

Rashim Bajaj's story is inspiring and showcases the challenges individuals face when dealing with unexplained infertility. Unexplained infertility, also known as idiopathic infertility, is a condition where couples cannot conceive naturally, and despite undergoing various infertility tests and diagnostic procedures, the cause remains unknown (*9 Inspiring Infertility Stories of Hope and Determination*, 2021). It can be a frustrating and emotionally distressing experience, as the couple is left without a clear explanation for their fertility struggles.

In Rashim's case, her journey began with a diagnosis of unexplained infertility, which led to failed IVF attempts and the suggestion of adoption as an option. However, she and her husband were determined to have a child of their own, and they refused to give up. They continued their quest to pinpoint the cause of their infertility and treat it.

After thorough research and consulting with a new doctor, they discovered that Rashim had tuberculosis in her reproductive system, which was previously overlooked. This finding provided a ray of hope, as they now had a specific issue to address rather than facing unexplained infertility (*9 Inspiring Infertility Stories of Hope and Determination*, 2021).

Rashim underwent treatment for tuberculosis and was also diagnosed with stage 3 endometriosis, which required surgery. Despite some complications during and after the surgery, she persevered. Her dedication and resilience paid off when she successfully became pregnant through IUI.

However, her pregnancy journey was not without challenges, including low placenta and gestational diabetes. Nevertheless, Rashim managed to carry her pregnancy to term and welcomed her first child into the world. In fact, she became pregnant for the second time, naturally this time. The happy couple were overjoyed by their complete family.

Rashim's story highlights the importance of persistence, proactive research, and seeking second opinions when dealing with unexplained infertility. It also emphasizes that miracles can happen for those who continue to demand and work toward their dreams of parenthood (*9 Inspiring Infertility Stories of Hope and Determination*, 2021).

In this chapter, we will explore the crucial steps that help prepare our bodies (and minds) for pregnancy. It all begins with setting goals for yourself as a future mother, for your husband, and for you both as a couple. The importance of nutrition, exercise, and weight management are often overlooked in our attempts to get pregnant. But it starts with laying the foundation for pregnancy. This means setting attainable goals to prioritize your well-being and pave the way for a healthy and joyful experience.

SETTING GOALS

Manifesting your desire for a child starts with creating that aura around your togetherness as a couple. This vibe will prompt you to want to make plans, and it is, in fact, the next logical step.

Make a Plan and Take Action

Parenthood is filled with dreams and aspirations. Just like you've set goals throughout your life, setting goals for pregnancy is equally important. Begin by discussing your plans with your partner and envisioning the kind of family you wish to create. Having a clear vision can be empowering and motivating (CDC, 2018).

See Your Doctor

Your healthcare provider is your ally on this journey. Before trying to conceive, schedule a preconception health checkup. This visit is a chance to discuss your health history, any existing medical conditions, and previous pregnancy experiences. Make a list of questions to ensure you cover everything important to you (CDC, 2018). Here are a few ideas about what to discuss in these crucial meetings with your healthcare provider.

- **Medical Conditions:** If you have any underlying medical conditions, work with your healthcare provider to manage and control them effectively. Conditions such as diabetes, high blood pressure, and thyroid disorders need special attention.
- **Lifestyle and Behaviors:** Openly discuss lifestyle factors with your doctors, including smoking, alcohol consumption, and exposure to toxic substances. They can provide guidance, counseling, and support services tailored to your needs.
- **Medications:** Review all medications you are currently taking, including prescriptions, over-the-counter drugs, supplements, and vitamins. Collaborate with your healthcare provider to determine the best approach for your health and your baby's well-being.
- **Vaccinations:** Ensure you are up to date with vaccinations recommended for pregnant individuals, such as the flu vaccine and Tdap. Staying protected against preventable diseases is essential for both you and your baby's health.

Folic Acid

Folic acid is a superhero in prenatal care. Start taking 400 micrograms of folic acid daily for at least one month before conceiving and throughout your pregnancy. This essential B vitamin helps prevent significant congenital disabilities of the baby's brain and spine –spina bifida is more common than you'd think it is (CDC, 2018).

Healthy Lifestyle Choices

Pregnancy is a time for positive changes. Commit to quitting smoking, abstaining from alcohol, and avoiding certain drugs. Seek support if needed, as these habits can negatively affect your pregnancy journey — low birth weight, fetal alcohol syndrome, and increased risk of miscarriage are some very real risks of making unhealthy lifestyle choices while trying to have a baby.

Avoid Toxic Substances and Environmental Contaminants

Create a safe environment for your growing family by identifying and avoiding harmful chemicals, pollutants, and toxic substances. Taking proactive steps now can protect your reproductive health (CDC, 2018).

Reach and Maintain a Healthy Weight

A healthy weight is the foundation for a smooth pregnancy. Prioritize balanced nutrition and regular physical activity as part of your daily life. If you're underweight or overweight, consult your doctor for guidance on achieving and maintaining a healthy weight (CDC, 2018).

Learn Your Family History

Family health history can hold valuable insights into potential genetic factors that might affect your pregnancy. Share this information with your healthcare provider to make informed decisions about your prenatal care (CDC, 2018).

Get Mentally Healthy

Mental well-being is essential during pregnancy. Prioritize your emotional health, and don't hesitate to seek help if you experience persistent feelings of anxiety, sadness, or stress. Your healthcare provider can support and guide you to ensure you feel your best throughout this transformative journey (CDC, 2018).

Preparing for pregnancy is a profound and life-altering journey that begins with setting clear goals and prioritizing your health and well-being. By taking these steps and working closely with your healthcare provider, you can create a nurturing and supportive environment for your future child. Embrace this chapter in your lives with love, positivity, and determination to provide the best possible start for your little one (CDC, 2018).

DIET

Embarking on the path to parenthood is a beautiful and transformative experience, but for some couples, the road to conception can be filled with unexpected challenges. While there are factors beyond our control regarding fertility, one aspect we can influence is our diet. Nutrition and maintaining a healthy body weight are crucial in the journey to parenthood for both women and men. Let's explore how the foods we choose can affect our fertility and increase our chances of conceiving (Kaufman, 2018).

Women and Fertility

Preparing your body for pregnancy is a significant step in your fertility journey. Maintaining a healthy weight and selecting the right foods can create an optimal environment for your baby's growth over the nine months of pregnancy. Focus on incorporating sources of essential nutrients, such as folic acid and iron, into your diet (Kaufman, 2018).

Men and Fertility

It is important to remember that fertility isn't just a concern for women. Men should also aim for a healthy body weight and balanced diet. Obesity in men can alter hormone levels and affect sperm count and motility. To support healthy sperm production, include plenty of fruits and vegetables in your diet, as they contain vitamins, minerals, and antioxidants that can enhance sperm quality (Kaufman, 2018).

Finding Your Healthy Weight

Maintaining a healthy weight is vital for both women and men seeking to conceive. Extreme weight fluctuations can disrupt hormone levels and interfere with ovulation. Women who are overweight or obese may benefit from weight loss to improve fertility, while those who are underweight might experience irregular menstrual cycles or ovulation issues (Kaufman, 2018). Finding a balanced approach to weight management is essential, avoiding fad diets that deprive your body of necessary nutrients. Seek guidance from a registered dietician nutritionist to develop a healthy eating plan tailored to your needs (Kaufman, 2018).

Include Adequate Iron

Iron plays a crucial role in fertility. Research from The Nurses' Health Study II suggests that a diet rich in vegetable-based iron sources and iron supplements may reduce the risk of ovulatory infertility. Vegetarian iron sources include beans, lentils, spinach, fortified cereals, whole grains, and vitamin C-rich foods like citrus fruits and berries can enhance iron absorption (Kaufman, 2018).

The "Fertility Diet" Pattern

In 2007, Harvard researchers introduced the "Fertility Diet" pattern (Kaufman, 2018). Women with ovulatory infertility who followed this eating pattern experienced a 66% lower risk of ovulatory infertility and a 27% reduced risk of infertility from other causes compared to those who didn't follow the diet closely. The key components of this diet include:

- Less trans fat and more monounsaturated fat (found in avocados and olive oil).
- Reduced animal protein and increased vegetable protein.
- Increased consumption of high-fiber, low-glycemic carbohydrate-rich foods (including whole grains).
- Greater reliance on vegetarian sources of iron over meat sources.
- Multivitamins.
- Preferential use of high-fat dairy over low-fat options.

Incorporate a variety of vegetables, opt for monounsaturated fats over saturated and trans fats, make at least half your grains whole, and ensure you get enough calcium-rich foods, including dairy, to meet your nutrient needs and maintain a healthy weight (Kaufman, 2018). Consider taking a good multivitamin supplement.

Folic Acid

If you're pregnant or planning to become pregnant, it's important to know about folic acid. It's a vital nutrient also known as folate or vitamin B9. Without it, your baby's healthy growth and development could be at risk. Folic acid is involved in several crucial processes during pregnancy, so ensure you're getting enough of it through your diet or supplements.

Folic acid helps prevent neural tube defects, which develop in the early stages of pregnancy, often before a woman knows she is pregnant. The U.S. Preventative Service Task Force recommends a daily supplement containing 400 to 800 micrograms of folic acid in addition to consuming folate and folic acid-rich foods like dark leafy greens and fortified grains (Kaufman, 2018).

The Role of Folic Acid in Pregnancy

Neural Tube Development:

Fun fact — did you know that consuming enough folic acid during pregnancy can be critical to your baby's health? This super nutrient can help prevent congenital disabilities or birth defects that can affect the brain, spine, or spinal cord. Ensuring you're getting enough folic acid before and during pregnancy can significantly lower the risk of these harmful conditions (*Folate and Pregnancy*, 2019). So, let's make sure you and your baby get all the benefits of this essential vitamin!

DNA Synthesis and Cell Growth:

During pregnancy, DNA synthesis and cell growth are vital processes that require the presence of folic acid

(*Folate and Pregnancy*, 2019). This nutrient is especially essential as the baby develops rapidly, facilitating the formation of new tissues and cells. Ensuring adequate intake of folic acid is crucial for maintaining the health and well-being of both the mother and the baby.

Red Blood Cell Formation:

Every expectant mother deserves the best care possible for her growing baby. That's why it's important to remember the vital role that folic acid plays in the production of red blood cells (*Folate and Pregnancy*, 2019). By ensuring the formation of healthy red blood cells, folic acid helps prevent anemia and ensures that the developing baby receives the necessary oxygen and nutrients for optimal growth and development.

Folic Acid-Rich Foods:

To ensure a sufficient intake of folic acid during pregnancy, it is essential to include foods rich in this vitamin in your diet (*Folate and Pregnancy*, 2019). Here are some excellent dietary sources of folic acid:

Leafy Greens:

Spinach, kale, collard greens, and other leafy vegetables are rich in folate (*Folate and Pregnancy* 2019). They can be incorporated into salads, smoothies, or cooked dishes.

Legumes:

Lentils, chickpeas, and black beans are excellent sources of folate (*Folate and Pregnancy*, 2019). They can be used in soups, stews, or as a side dish.

Fortified Foods:

Many breakfast cereals, bread, and pasta are fortified with folic acid (*Folate and Pregnancy*, 2019). Check the labels for added folate to ensure you're getting enough.

Citrus Fruits:

Oranges, grapefruits, and their juices contain moderate amounts of folate (*Folate and Pregnancy*, 2019). They can be enjoyed as a refreshing and healthy snack.

Avocado:

Avocado is a nutrient-rich fruit that provides a decent amount of folate (*Folate and Pregnancy*, 2019). It can be used in salads, sandwiches, or as a topping.

Asparagus:

Asparagus is a seasonal vegetable that is a good source of folate (*Folate and Pregnancy*, 2019). It can be grilled, roasted, or added to various dishes.

Folic acid is a critical nutrient for a healthy pregnancy and the baby's well-being. Ensuring an adequate intake of folate-rich foods and, if necessary, taking a folic acid supplement as recommended by your healthcare provider can help reduce the risk of congenital disabilities and support your child's healthy development. Prioritizing this essential nutrient during pregnancy is a simple yet powerful way to give your baby the best start in life.

Always consult your healthcare provider before starting any dietary supplement. Consider consulting a registered dietitian nutritionist who can help you navigate this important chapter in your life. Remember, nourishing your body is a loving step toward welcoming a new life into your family.

EXERCISE

While fertility can be influenced by various factors, one crucial element that plays a significant role in the path to conception is exercise. Both women and men can benefit from incorporating regular physical activity into their lives as they embark on the beautiful journey of creating a family. Exercise has a direct bearing on fertility in a few ways.

Exercise and Fertility for Women

I know that when you're caught up in the rat race of the humdrum daily grind, it seems like there is never enough time to do the things you know are important, but we tend to treat it as an optional afterthought. However, one of the most integral parts of your fertility action plan has to be exercise, and here is why (*The Benefits of Exercising*, n.d.).

Boosting Fertility

Regular, moderate exercise has been shown to enhance fertility in women. Engaging in physical activity that raises your heart rate, makes you breathe faster, and induces a feeling of warmth can increase the chances of getting pregnant. This doesn't mean you need to become a gym enthusiast; activities as simple as brisk walking can be considered moderate exercise.

Healthy Body Weight

Exercise contributes to maintaining a healthy body weight, a critical factor in fertility. Extreme weight fluctuations can disrupt hormone levels and affect ovulation. For women who are overweight or obese, losing weight through exercise can improve fertility. Conversely, underweight women may experience irregular menstrual cycles or ovulation issues and can benefit from exercise to reach a healthier BMI.

Mental Health Benefits

Exercise not only benefits physical health but also mental well-being. Planning for pregnancy can be both exciting and stressful. Staying active can help reduce stress, anxiety, and the risk of depression, creating a positive mindset for the journey ahead.

Health Benefits for Babies

Maintaining an active lifestyle during pregnancy extends benefits to your child's long-term health. Children born to active parents are more likely to adopt an active lifestyle themselves, promoting their well-being.

Exercise and Fertility for Men

Male fertility can be vastly improved through regular exercise. Here are some of how exercise affects fertility in men (*The Benefits of Exercising*, n.d.).

Supporting Sperm Quality

Men, too, can reap the rewards of exercise when it comes to fertility. Regular physical activity can contribute to healthier sperm quality, making it a valuable factor for couples aiming to conceive.

Healthy Body Weight

Maintaining a healthy body weight is not only important for women but also for men. Being overweight can affect the quantity and quality of sperm, emphasizing the importance of regular exercise to manage weight.

Exercise and IVF

For couples undergoing IVF treatment, exercise remains an essential component of overall health. While moderate exercise is generally considered safe and beneficial, individuals who engage in intense or vigorous exercise may be advised to reduce their activity levels during IVF treatment, especially if the treatment is focused on addressing ovulation issues (*The Benefits of Exercising*, n.d.).

Exercise and Low BMI

It's important to note that low body mass index (BMI) due to excessive exercise and inadequate calorie intake can impact fertility negatively. For women struggling to conceive and experiencing irregular periods or amenorrhea (absence of periods), reducing intense exercise to a moderate level while ensuring sufficient calorie intake may help improve fertility (*The Benefits of Exercising*, n.d.).

For these reasons that exercise is a valuable tool for both women and men on their fertility journey. Regular, moderate physical activity can enhance the chances of conception, promote a healthy pregnancy, and contribute to a positive mental outlook during this transformative period. Whether you're planning to start a family or are undergoing fertility treatment, maintaining a balanced and active lifestyle can make a significant difference in your path to parenthood. It is a shared journey that begins with taking steps toward a healthier, more active future for both you and your partner (*The Benefits of Exercising*, n.d.).

WEIGHT

A crucial factor influencing fertility that often gets overlooked is body weight. Achieving and maintaining a healthy weight can significantly impact your chances of conceiving and experiencing a successful pregnancy. In this section, we explore the profound link between fertility and weight, shedding light on why proper weight management is essential for those aspiring to start a family (Skiadas, 2023).

Determining a Healthy Weight

Before delving into the effects of weight on fertility, it is essential to understand how to assess how healthy you are in terms of your body weight. A straightforward method is calculating your body mass index (BMI), for which the Centers for Disease Control and Prevention provides a convenient calculator (Skiadas, 2023). To calculate your BMI, simply convert your weight to kilograms (kg) and height to meters; divide your weight by your height squared.

For example, if you weigh 65 kg (143.3 lbs) and are 1.68 m (around five feet five inches) tall, you work out your BMI by squaring your height: 1.68 x 1.68 = 2.82. Then divide 65 by 2.82 = 23.04. Therefore, your BMI would be 23.0. This would fall into the normal category.

- Normal: BMI between 19 and 24

- Underweight: BMI less than 19
- Overweight: BMI between 25 and 29
- Obese: BMI greater than 30

If, like me, math isn't your strong suit, check out the various online BMI calculators to do the math for you.

How Obesity Impacts Fertility

Obesity can substantially affect fertility, primarily through its impact on ovulation — the process in which an egg is released from the ovaries. Obesity can seriously hinder fertility (Skiadas, 2023):

- **Irregular Menstrual Cycles:** Obesity often leads to irregular menstrual cycles or the absence of periods altogether, making it challenging to determine the timing of ovulation. Without ovulation, pregnancy becomes impossible.
- **Hormonal Imbalances:** Obesity can disrupt hormones, causing the body to stop producing estrogen. Hormonal imbalances further complicate the process of ovulation.
- **Associated Health Conditions:** Obesity is often accompanied by health issues like thyroid disease, insulin resistance, and diabetes, all of which can negatively affect fertility.

How Being Underweight Affects Fertility

Being underweight can also lead to fertility problems, primarily due to ovulatory dysfunction.

- *Hormone Disruption*: Underweight women who exercise excessively or have a low caloric intake may experience hormone disruptions, leading to estrogen deficiency. This can result in irregular menstrual cycles or amenorrhea (the absence of periods).
- *Pregnancy Complications*: It is important to note that underweight women who do become pregnant face higher risks of miscarriage, premature birth, and delivering babies with low birth weight.

The Impact of Weight on Male Fertility

Obesity in men can lead to significant changes in testosterone levels and other reproductive hormones. Additionally, overweight and obese men often have lower sperm counts and reduced sperm motility compared to those with a normal BMI.

Seeking Guidance for Weight Management

If you're contemplating pregnancy and find yourself either underweight or overweight, it is crucial to consult your healthcare provider. They can help you identify any underlying medical conditions and offer guidance on weight management. Your provider may also suggest connecting with a fertility specialist or a weight management expert to create a personalized plan for your journey toward parenthood (Skiadas, 2023).

The profound connection between fertility and weight underscores the importance of proper weight management for anyone hoping to start a family. Whether you are looking to shed excess weight or gain it, remember that achieving and maintaining a healthy weight can significantly enhance your chances of conception and a successful pregnancy. Embrace the journey with a holistic perspective, envisioning a future filled with the joys of parenthood, knowing that support is available every step of the way (Skiadas, 2023).

Once our bodies and minds are perfectly aligned with our goals, the next step is to become more deliberate in optimizing our chances of conceiving. You would be surprised how a few little tricks can help improve your chances of success.

4

EMBARKING ON PARENTHOOD— CONCEPTION OPTIMIZATION

"My husband and I embarked on our journey to start a family right after our wedding in 2010, both of us being 25 years old at the time. However, as months passed, I started to have this unsettling feeling that the gift of parenthood might elude us. Call it intuition or a self-fulfilling prophecy, but unfortunately, my initial fears proved to be right.

The eight years that followed were an emotional roller-coaster, unlike anything I had ever experienced. It's hard to put into words the depth of the emotions I went through. A profound and perpetual sadness seemed to engulf me—a constant companion on my life's journey.

Each passing year seemed to add to the weight of despair. Every negative pregnancy test, each failed IVF attempt, every baby shower I attended, and every pregnancy announcement I heard chipped away at my spirit. It wasn't that I couldn't be happy for others; it was a stark reminder of the void within me, making me feel like my body had failed me.

With increasing bitterness, I discovered that my heart could break multiple times, each time more painful than the last, especially when my second IVF cycle failed. But just before my third attempt, I made a conscious shift toward gratitude and positivity. I redirected my thoughts from what wasn't happening to what I desired to happen. I rewrote my narrative, transitioning from 'I can't get pregnant' to 'I can't wait to get pregnant.' The journey was far from easy, but I was determined to change my mindset and outlook.

Finally, in 2018, after our third IVF cycle, I received the news I had been yearning for. I vividly recall taking a digital pregnancy test, and the word 'pregnant' appeared on the screen. After years of seeing 'not pregnant,' it felt surreal, a moment etched in my memory forever. We welcomed a beautiful baby boy into our lives in January 2019.

Fast forward to 2020, a decade after my journey began, I found the strength to share my story. Infertility often carries with it a sense of shame and embarrassment, particularly in South Asian cultures. By opening up about my experience, I hope to chip away at the stigma surrounding infertility. I also aspire to offer a ray of hope to those who, like me, once felt broken, hopeless, and desperate. Remember, there is hope, even in the darkest of times.

With warmth,

Saira, UK (*I Changed My Narrative from "I Can't Get Pregnant" to "I Can't Wait to Get Pregnant,"* 2020)

THE BEST TIMES FOR CONCEPTION

Now, let's get down to the nitty-gritty of how to get the baby-making magic started. First, let's talk about the best time to sprinkle a little stardust into your life!

They say the magic window for baby-making is usually about 12–16 days before your expected period (Robinson, 2022). But hold up, don't set your calendar in stone just yet because nailing down the exact moment when Mother Nature decides to do her thing can be a bit tricky. We're all unique, after all!

One cool trick is tracking your morning temperature, aka your basal body temperature. Grab yourself a fancy basal body thermometer, and every morning, before even getting out of bed, take your temp (Robinson, 2022). When you notice a slight, steady rise that sticks around until your next period, that's a sign that ovulation has probably happened. So, you can kind of predict when it might swing by in future cycles.

Then there are these nifty tools called ovulation predictor kits (OPKs). They detect a hormone called LH, which tends to skyrocket 24–48 hours before you pop that egg (Robinson, 2022). You can go with the old-school test strips or the fancier digital monitors. They're handy for precision but not always 100% spot-on.

Now, if you're all about tech, there are apps for everything these days, including tracking your cycle. You pop in details like the first day of your period, OPK results, and your temperature. These apps even shoot you reminders when you're likely to be super fertile (Robinson, 2022). But a heads up: many assume a textbook 28-day cycle, which isn't everyone's rhythm.

For those who want to go full high-tech, there are fertility monitors. They're like little wizards that use test strips and a digital monitor to measure LH and estrogen levels, finding your prime baby-making days and saving the info for later (Robinson, 2022). Just remember, they can be a bit pricey and may assume a standard cycle length.

Now, if you're feeling all-natural, you can go with the cervical mucus method. It's all about checking your vaginal mucus. "Wet days" are the golden ticket, with clear, slippery mucus that's kind of like egg whites (Robinson, 2022). That's when the baby dance is most likely to be a success.

When it comes to timing, experts suggest getting cozy as close to ovulation as you can. Some say go for it every day starting five days before the big O and keep the party going for one more day afterward. Others advise that you keep it low-key with a "no-pressure" every-other-day rendezvous (Robinson, 2022).

But here's the bottom line: this baby-making journey can be a rollercoaster of emotions, so don't forget to keep your chin up and stay positive. If you're not seeing a plus sign on that pregnancy test after six months, it's all good! It's just time to give a shout-out to a medical pro who can offer some guidance and support.

TRACKING OVULATION AND FERTILITY SIGNS

What Is Fertility Awareness?

Fertility awareness, also known as fertility tracking, ovulation tracking, or natural family planning, is all about getting to know your body and its natural rhythm (*Methods for Tracking Your Fertility and Ovulation*, 2020). It's like getting the inside scoop on when your ovaries are gearing up to release an egg—a crucial piece of the baby-making puzzle.

The Benefits of Fertility Tracking

Okay, so here's the scoop: There are only about six days in your entire month when pregnancy is on the table. Clinical wisdom tells us that these prime days fall between day 10 and day 17 in a typical 28-day cycle. But guess what? Mother Nature doesn't always play by the rules. Studies have shown that ovulation can be as unpredictable as the weather, and things like stress, diet, and even sleep can throw a curveball into your cycle.

This is where fertility awareness-based methods (FABMs) swoop in to save the day. Your body dishes out little signs throughout your menstrual cycle, like breadcrumbs leading you to the treasure (that treasure being the fertile days).

When used correctly, FABMs are about 76–88% accurate in nailing down your fertile window. And here's the secret sauce: combining different methods can make them even more effective. Teamwork makes the dream work, right?

Common Signs of Ovulation

Want to know if you're in the fertility zone? Keep an eye out for these signs:

- a positive result on an ovulation predictor test
- a sustained rise in your basal body temperature (BBT)
- cervical mucus that's like the consistency of egg whites (no joke!)
- a saliva ferning pattern (yes, your spit can give you clues)
- changes in your cervical position
- a little thing called Mittelschmerz pain (ovulating pain)
- increased libido (hubba-hubba)

- tender breasts (*Methods for Tracking Your Fertility and Ovulation*, 2020)

Fertility Awareness-Based Methods You Can Use

Now, let's talk about methods! There's more than one way to track your fertility (*Methods for Tracking Your Fertility and Ovulation*, 2020):

- **Calendar Method (Standard Days Method):** Predict your fertile days based on your cycle length and past period dates.
- **Basal Body Temperature Method:** Measures your morning temperature to detect shifts that signal ovulation.
- **Cervical Mucus Method:** Monitors changes in your cervical mucus throughout your cycle.
- **TwoDay Method®:** A variation of the cervical mucus method based on daily secretions.
- **Symptothermal Method (STM):** Combines BBT, cervical mucus, and calendar methods for super accuracy.
- **Cervical Position Method:** Tracks changes in your cervix's firmness, openness, and position.
- **Ovulation Predictor Kits:** Test your urine for a surge in LH.
- **Saliva Ferning Tests:** Check for fern-like crystals in your dried saliva.

Apps That Make Fertility Tracking a Breeze

Don't worry; you don't need a detective's notebook to track it all. There are tons of apps to help you stay on top of your fertility game (*Methods for Tracking Your Fertility and Ovulation*, 2020):

- **Fertility Friend:** Offers a variety of tracking features and a supportive community.
- **Natural Cycles:** An FDA-cleared birth control app that predicts your fertile window.
- **Glow:** A comprehensive app with health insights and partner-sharing options.
- **Kindara:** Let you track an impressive range of data, from BBT to moods.
- **Modern Fertility:** Predicts your two most fertile days and even scans ovulation test results.

Other Fertility Tracking Gadgets and Tools

Feeling a bit tech-savvy? Check out these cool gadgets (*Methods for Tracking Your Fertility and Ovulation*, 2020):

- **Ava:** A bracelet that tracks various body signals to pinpoint your fertile days.
- **OvuSense:** A sensor you insert overnight that predicts ovulation with 99% accuracy.
- **Priya (Coming Soon):** A ring-shaped device that continuously measures your core body temperature.

So, there you have it! A sneak peek into the wonderful world of fertility awareness. Remember, your journey to parenthood is uniquely yours, and these tools are here to help you along the way. If you ever need a helping hand or some expert advice, don't hesitate to reach out to a healthcare professional.

STRATEGIES FOR ENHANCING FERTILITY DURING INTERCOURSE

The subject of conception can be difficult. The success of a relationship is determined by several factors, including each person's health and the timing of their decision to have a child. But, in the end, conception is all about sex. There is no way his sperm will ever get into contact with your egg without it (or assistance from a lab).

So, are there any positions that improve the chances of conception? Is there a specific time when you should begin? Here are some ideas to assist you in maximizing your sex life to produce children (HealthyWomen Editors, 2014).

Be Punctual

When attempting to conceive, timing is everything. The "fertility window," which lasts from five days before ovulation to the day you ovulate, is the best period to conceive. You are most fertile two days before and on the day of ovulation.

It's tough to estimate when you'll ovulate because it depends on how long your menstrual cycle is and whether it's constant from month to month. Determine the day of your next period, then subtract 14 days as a general rule (HealthyWomen Editors, 2014). Or use a free online fertility calculator.

Do It Regularly

While ovulation is crucial, you don't want to restrict sex to your fertile window. While having sex once a day in the days preceding ovulation can be beneficial, you should ideally have sex every few days throughout the month to increase your chances of hitting the fertility jackpot (HealthyWomen Editors, 2014). Basically, have sex whenever you want and pay special attention to the days when you're most likely to get pregnant.

Find a Good Position

Regarding how you should have sex, there is no scientific proof that one position is more likely to result in pregnancy than another (HealthyWomen Editors, 2014). Women have become pregnant from various situations, but you can boost your chances by ensuring a few requirements are satisfied.

First, you want your partner's sperm to go as close to your cervix as possible, which requires deep penetration. According to research, missionary and doggy-style allow the penis to reach the recesses at the front and back of the cervix (HealthyWomen Editors, 2014).

Second, you want to make it as easy for the sperm to reach your egg as possible, which means they shouldn't be fighting gravity. Avoid postures such as "lady on top" and "standing up." After sex, it may be beneficial to lie down for up to 30 minutes to ensure that no ejaculate spills out (HealthyWomen Editors, 2014). Some ladies additionally place a pillow beneath their lower back to tilt their pelvis up slightly.

Don't Worry About Having an Orgasm (But Try Anyway!)

When you're attempting to conceive, your man's orgasm is the most important (HealthyWomen Editors, 2014). Don't feel obligated to orgasm before your guy, but you should aim to get there for the sheer pleasure of it! Having fun and feeling good will only improve sex and make conception simpler.

Given that trying to conceive kind of turns the excitement of intimacy into a chore and can affect the mood in the boudoir significantly, communication, relaxation, and fun are prerequisites to having a great time. Try not to allow becoming pregnant to become a pressure trigger or stressor, as this could intensify any pre-existing infertility issues each of you might be struggling with (even if you are not aware of them yet). Both male and female infertility need closer examination, but we should start with female infertility first.

Make a Difference with Your Review
Embrace the Power of Sharing

"Your words have the potential to change lives. Use them wisely."

— UNKNOWN

Hello there,

I want to share a story with you. It's a story of hope, empowerment, and the dream of parenthood. This story is found within the pages of "Navigating the Fertility Maze," a book that's meant to be a guiding light for those on their fertility journey.

Now, I'm reaching out to ask for your support in sharing this story and the valuable knowledge it contains. But it's not just any support; it's a gift of kindness that costs you nothing but a few moments of your time.

Imagine someone you've never met. They're standing at the beginning of their fertility journey, feeling a mix of emotions - hope, uncertainty, and perhaps a touch of fear. They need guidance, knowledge, and encouragement, and your review can provide just that.

Would you help this person, even if you never got credit for it?

You have the opportunity to be a guiding star for them, to offer insights that can change their lives forever. Your review could help...

...one more couple find the information they need to start their journey.
...one more individual gain confidence in their fertility choices.
...one more dream of parenthood come to life.

It takes less than 60 seconds to leave a review. Simply scan the QR code below:

If you're someone who believes in the power of sharing knowledge, empathy, and support, then you're the kind of person who can make a real difference in someone's life.

You're not just a reader; you're part of a community of caring individuals.

By supporting this person on their journey, you're also helping us achieve our mission of making fertility knowledge accessible to all. It's a mission that we're deeply passionate about, and your review is a vital part of that effort.

Thank you from the bottom of our hearts for considering this request. We appreciate your kindness and your willingness to help others.

Your biggest supporter, Kasia Marshall

PS - If you know someone who could benefit from this book, consider sharing it with them. Your generosity could be the spark that lights their path to parenthood. Sharing is caring, after all.

5

SILENT STRUGGLES—FEMALE INFERTILITY

"From childhood, I longed to be a mother. I played with baby dolls, sang lullabies, and even changed pretend diapers. My path led me to become a nurse, specializing in caring for mothers and babies. But as life would have it, the one thing that didn't come naturally was my journey to motherhood.

My husband, Brandon, and I embarked on the path to parenthood after three years of marriage, believing we had it all figured out. We saved, planned meticulously, and eagerly awaited the moment we'd become a family. However, months turned into more months, and frustration crept in. I tracked every cycle, monitored my basal body temperature religiously at 6 a.m., and peed on countless ovulation strips, all leading to another negative pregnancy test.

As a nurse specializing in maternity care, I felt broken. I witnessed the joy of countless families welcoming babies while my struggle intensified. Friends and family questioned why we hadn't conceived, oblivious to our relentless efforts.

Around the 15-month mark, we met Dr. Albert Hsu at MU Health Care. His hopeful smile and reassurances breathed new life into us. We had a plan, and finally a glimmer of hope.

I underwent procedures, blood draws, and started Letrozole. Nervous but determined, I took the medication. And then, the moment of truth arrived—a positive pregnancy test. Tears of joy flowed.

However, our journey took an unexpected turn at our first ultrasound. The technician's silence spoke volumes—two empty amniotic sacs. Two weeks of agonizing uncertainty followed until we faced the heartbreaking reality—our babies hadn't grown.

Amid the pain, faith in God sustained us. We embraced the path to healing and tried again. The Letrozole worked its magic, and this time, a smiling ultrasound technician unveiled a thriving baby. On June 4, 2019, after two and a half years of unwavering hope, Owen Michael entered our lives. His arrival filled our hearts with a love like no other." —Lyndsay Kalista (*Fertility Is a Journey*, 2021).

Lyndsay's story was undoubtedly heart-wrenching, with a joyous, happy ending. For some, the journey to parenthood is pretty smooth, while others struggle down a path fraught with pain and uncertainty. However, every journey must start somewhere, and understanding the captivating journey from the release of a mature egg to that incredible moment of conception is a good starting point.

Imagine each step in the intricate dance of human reproduction as a key to unlocking the magic of life. This dance is a harmonious symphony, where every move must be executed flawlessly for the grand finale—a new life.

However, facing the challenges of getting pregnant head-on by understanding its causes is where our journey truly starts to take off.

THE DANCE OF CONCEPTION: A PRECISE CHOREOGRAPHY

Picture this: one of your ovaries releases a mature egg, a tiny traveler embarking on a remarkable journey. It is gently picked up by the fallopian tube, where it eagerly awaits its partner—sperm. These determined swimmers, having traversed the cervix, navigated the uterus, and embarked on a mission through the fallopian tube, finally meet their destiny—the egg. This enchanting encounter results in fertilization (Mayo Clinic, 2018).

Now, the fertilized egg launches its odyssey. As a zygote, it travels down the fallopian tube, transforming into a morula and then a blastocyst. This intrepid blastocyst arrives at its ultimate destination, the cozy lining of the uterus. Here, it firmly attaches itself in a process known as implantation, preparing to grow and thrive (Mayo Clinic, 2018).

The Masterpiece of Creation: The Female Reproductive System

To understand infertility, it's vital to appreciate the intricate symphony that is the female reproductive system. This symphony is composed of five key players: the ovaries, fallopian tubes, uterus, cervix, and vagina, collectively orchestrating the magical journey of conception.

THE CAUSES OF FEMALE INFERTILITY

Now that we've established what the various instruments in this orchestra are, we can delve into the causes of discord that result in tears along the way. Female infertility can arise from multiple sources, each affecting a different stage of the process.

Ovulation Disorders: The Dance of the Egg

Imagine the egg as the star of the show. Problems with ovulation, where this star doesn't take center stage as often as it should, account for a significant portion of infertility cases. Factors such as hormonal imbalances, disruptions in the regulation of reproductive hormones, or issues in the ovaries can lead to ovulation disorders. Here are some key culprits (Mayo Clinic, 2018):

- **PCOS:** This hormonal imbalance disrupts ovulation and is associated with insulin resistance, obesity, and other symptoms.
- **Hypothalamic Dysfunction:** Physical or emotional stress, fluctuations in body weight, or even recent substantial weight changes can disrupt the hormones responsible for ovulation.
- **Primary Ovarian Insufficiency:** This condition, usually linked to autoimmune responses or genetic factors, results in premature ovarian failure, lowering estrogen production.

Tubal Troubles: The Path Blocked

The fallopian tubes, like bridges in our dance, facilitate the egg's journey to meet the sperm. However, damage or blockages in these vital passageways can create significant obstacles. Common causes of tubal infertility include (Mayo Clinic, 2018):

- **Pelvic Inflammatory Disease (PID):** Infections like chlamydia and gonorrhea can lead to inflammation of the uterus and fallopian tubes, causing blockages.

- **Previous Abdominal or Pelvic Surgery:** Surgical history, including procedures for ectopic pregnancies, can disrupt the fallopian tubes' function.
- **Endometriosis:** When uterine tissue grows outside the uterus, it can lead to scarring and blockages in the fallopian tubes.

Uterine or Cervical Challenges: Preparing the Stage

The implantation stage must be perfectly set. Issues within the uterus or cervix can disrupt this crucial process or increase the risk of miscarriage. Some factors to consider include (Mayo Clinic, 2018):

- **Benign Polyps or Tumors:** While common, these uterine growths can sometimes interfere with fertility, though many women with them still manage to conceive.
- **Congenital Uterine Issues:** Some women may have a uterus with an unusual shape, which can affect pregnancy.
- **Cervical Stenosis:** Narrowing of the cervix, whether due to genetics or damage, can create obstacles.
- **Cervical Mucus:** The cervix must produce the right type of mucus to allow sperm to travel into the uterus.

The Enigma: Unexplained Infertility

In some cases, the puzzle of infertility remains unsolved. A blend of minor factors in both parents can lead to unexplained fertility issues. While it can be frustrating, remember that sometimes this problem can resolve itself with time. However, it's essential not to delay seeking treatment (Mayo Clinic, 2018).

DIAGNOSING AND ASSESSING FERTILITY ISSUES

If you've been having regular unprotected sex without conceiving, experts recommend considering an infertility evaluation after a year if you're under 35 years old or after six months if you're over 35. If you're over 40, it's best to talk to your obstetrician-gynecologist (ob-gyn) right away about an evaluation (*Evaluating Infertility*, 2020).

Who Performs Infertility Evaluations?

Your ob-gyn will usually be your first stop for an initial assessment. You may also consult with a reproductive endocrinologist or an ob-gyn with specialized training in infertility (*Evaluating Infertility*, 2020). Men might need to see a urologist. The key is to find a specialist you feel comfortable with.

What to Expect During Your First Visit to a Fertility Specialist

Your initial visit to a fertility specialist will involve a detailed medical history review and physical examination. Questions about menstrual cycles, pelvic issues, and reproductive disorders will be asked. Both you and your partner will be questioned about health concerns, medications, illnesses, birth defects or congenital disabilities in your family, past pregnancies, substance use, and sexual history (*Evaluating Infertility*, 2020).

Tests for Infertility

Infertility tests include laboratory tests, imaging tests, and certain procedures. These aim to examine reproductive organs and how they function. Laboratory tests often involve blood or semen samples.

Basic Testing for Men

Now, let's talk about the guys. Male fertility depends on healthy sperm production and their successful journey to meet the egg. Tests for men aim to uncover issues in this process (*Evaluating Infertility*, 2020):

- **Semen Analysis:** Yep, that means providing a sperm sample. It's usually collected by, well, self-help or stopping in mid-action during intercourse. A lab then checks the sample to evaluate sperm health.

- **Hormone Testing:** This involves a simple blood test to check hormone levels, especially testosterone.
- **Genetic Testing:** Sometimes, infertility may be linked to genetic factors, so genetic testing could be on the table.
- **Testicular Biopsy:** This one's rarer. It involves removing a tiny bit of testicle tissue for a closer look under a microscope. It helps identify issues with sperm production or blockages.
- **Imaging:** In some cases, ultrasounds or MRI scans might be needed to spot problems in the reproductive organs.

Basic Testing for Women

Now, let's shift the focus to the ladies. Female fertility relies on various factors, including egg health and a clear path for the egg to meet sperm. Women may undergo blood and urine tests, including those to determine ovulation, thyroid function, prolactin levels, and ovarian reserve (egg supply). Imaging procedures may include ultrasounds, sonohysterography, hysterosalpingography, hysteroscopy, and laparoscopy, depending on your symptoms and earlier test results.

- **Ovulation Testing:** A blood test to check hormone levels and confirm whether you're ovulating.

- **Thyroid Function Test:** If there's a suspicion of thyroid-related fertility issues, this blood test comes into play.
- **Hysterosalpingography:** A bit of a tongue-twister, but it's essential. This procedure checks the condition of the uterus and fallopian tube by injecting a special dye and taking an X-ray to help rule out any blockages in the fallopian tubes.
- **Ovarian Reserve Testing:** This assesses the number of eggs available for ovulation, usually starting with hormone tests early in your menstrual cycle.
- **Other Hormone Tests:** These keep an eye on various hormones that play a role in fertility.
- **Imaging:** Pelvic ultrasounds and sonohysterograms might be used to examine the uterus and ovaries in detail.

In some rare cases, more invasive procedures like hysteroscopy or laparoscopy might be necessary to diagnose and treat certain issues (Mayo Clinic, 2021).

Tracking Basal Body Temperature (BBT)

BBT tracking can confirm ovulation. A woman's temperature rises around ovulation and tracking it can help identify fertile days.

Urine Test

Urine tests can determine ovulation by detecting a surge in LH, indicating that ovulation will occur in the next 24 to 48 hours.

Progesterone Testing

Progesterone testing measures blood levels about one week before an expected period to confirm ovulation.

In most cases, infertility evaluations can be completed within a few menstrual cycles (*Evaluating Infertility*, 2020).

Some insurance plans may cover the cost of infertility evaluations. It is advisable to contact your insurance company to confirm coverage before embarking on your evaluation (*Evaluating Infertility*, 2020).

In the realm of fertility challenges, diagnosing and assessing infertility is the crucial first step on the path to parenthood. We've explored the various facets of this journey, from understanding when to consider an evaluation to the multitude of tests and procedures available for both women and men. It's a process that calls for patience, compassion, and perseverance.

Fertility can be influenced by a myriad of factors, including age, lifestyle, and pre-existing health conditions. For many, it may feel like an isolating struggle, but remember, you're not alone. Millions of couples worldwide have encountered similar challenges and have ultimately achieved their dream of parenthood.

As you embark on your journey, it's essential to find healthcare professionals you trust and feel comfortable with, as they will guide you through the intricacies of infertility testing. These experts can provide invaluable support and options tailored to your specific circumstances.

Now that we've unraveled the mysteries of infertility diagnosis, we'll dive into the world of Assisted Reproductive Technologies (ART) in the next chapter. ART offers a beacon of hope for couples facing fertility issues, providing innovative solutions to overcome the obstacles on the path to conception.

6

SCIENCE AND HOPE UNITE— EXPLORING ART

DAVINA AND BARRY: TRIUMPH OVER INFERTILITY

"Our infertility was a long and heart-wrenching one. Much like the stories of countless couples navigating this challenging path. We faced multiple miscarriages and battled the financial burden of fertility diagnostics and treatments without insurance support, grappled with strained family and social relationships, and, at times, felt like we were losing ourselves in the process.

We spared no effort in seeking intervention within our means, from counseling to less complex fertility treatments and even surgeries. We meticulously avoided anything that could pose a threat to our fertility, but despite our unwavering determination, success remained elusive.

Eventually, our journey led us to Massachusetts, where we discovered a way to access the fertility care we so desperately needed. This is where we found hope in the form of Dr. Brian Berger at Boston IVF. Under his compassionate and expert care, our lives were forever changed for the better. We were blessed with the arrival of our two beautiful children, Bella and Brennan.

However, our story didn't conclude with our own success. It took a new direction, one driven by a deep commitment to helping others facing the challenges of infertility. I became a passionate advocate, lobbying for infertility legislation both regionally and nationally. I collaborated with legislators, employers, and insurers to effect policy changes related to infertility benefits. Witnessing how a single voice could make an impactful difference, I went on to establish a nonprofit organization called 'Fertility Within Reach.' Its mission is to empower and educate individuals, equipping them with the tools needed to effectively advocate for fertility health benefits.

As we celebrate our journey through infertility, we are reminded that every success story carries the potential to inspire and uplift others. Boston IVF and Dr. Berger didn't just help create our family; they nurtured the spirit of a relentless advocate," (*Multiple Miscarriages*, 2023).

IVF

What Is IVF?

IVF is a nothing-short-of-miraculous medical process that has given numerous couples throughout the world happiness and hope. Infertility problems, which are commonly diagnosed when a couple is unable to conceive after a year of unprotected sexual activity, can be resolved by IVF (Ho, 2023).

This remarkable process involves uniting a person's eggs and sperm outside the body within a laboratory setting. The fertilized eggs, known as embryos, are then introduced into the uterus with the goal of achieving a successful pregnancy.

For individuals and couples who have suffered from various fertility issues, IVF can be a lifesaver. Although it has a lot of potential, it's crucial to comprehend the difficulties, expenses, and factors involved (Ho, 2023).

Who Should Consider IVF?

IVF is not a one-size-fits-all solution, and its appropriateness varies depending on individual circumstances (Ho, 2023). Here are some scenarios in which IVF might be a viable option:

- **Blocked or Absent Fallopian Tubes:** Since IVF avoids the use of these channels in conception, it can be a lifesaver for people with blocked or absent fallopian tubes.

- **"Male Factor Infertility:"** In cases where sperm counts or motility are low, or if sperm needs surgical extraction from the testicles, IVF can overcome these challenges.
- **Other Causes of Infertility:** If other infertility treatments have not yielded results, IVF may be the next logical step.
- **Advanced Maternal Age:** Women aged 40 or older who are keen to maximize their chances of pregnancy might opt for IVF.
- **Genetic Disease Prevention:** Couples with inherited genetic diseases may choose IVF coupled with PGT to ensure that embryos free from these diseases are implanted.
- **Ovarian Insufficiency:** When the ovaries stop producing eggs prematurely, IVF using donor eggs from another person may be an option.
- **Donor Sperm or Embryo:** Single females, female couples, or those facing specific fertility challenges might choose IVF with donor sperm or embryos.
- **Gestational Carrier:** In cases where pregnancy is impossible or unsafe for the individual or couple, such as those with health conditions, single males, or male couples, gestational carriers can be employed.

It's important to remember that while IVF holds tremendous potential, it's not without its disadvantages. These include:

- substantial costs
- potential side effects of injectable fertility medications and invasive procedures or increased risk of multiple gestations (twins or triplets)
- ovarian hyperstimulation syndrome if multiple embryos are transferred.

Some pregnancy complications, such as hypertensive disorders and preterm birth, may also be more common following IVF. Ectopic pregnancies, while less common than with other fertility treatments, can still occur.

It's advisable to explore less expensive and less invasive infertility treatments first, as several cycles of these treatments are often recommended before considering IVF.

How Does IVF Work?

IVF is a multi-step process that unfolds over several weeks. It is essential to understand what each stage entails (Ho, 2023).

- **Education:** Before embarking on the IVF journey, individuals (and their partners, if applicable) undergo thorough education. This covers the intricate steps involved, the potential risks and benefits of IVF, and guidance on self-administering injections at home.

- **Ovarian Stimulation:** The first step usually involves the administration of fertility medications to stimulate the ovaries. The goal is to produce multiple ovarian follicles, each containing an egg or oocyte. The specific medication regimen depends on the underlying cause of infertility and the protocols followed by the IVF center.
- **Ovarian Stimulation Without Medication:** In some cases, IVF can be performed without ovarian stimulation, a method known as "natural cycle IVF." This approach typically yields fewer eggs, and as a result, it's less commonly used worldwide.
- **FSH Injections:** FSH injections are a common component of ovarian stimulation. They encourage the growth of egg follicles. These injections are typically self-administered once daily, often in the evening, and can be given subcutaneously (under the skin).
- **Monitoring:** Regular pelvic ultrasounds and blood tests are performed during the stimulation phase. These tests assess follicle growth and hormone levels. Depending on the results, the FSH dosage may be adjusted.
- **GnRH Antagonists:** In some cases, GnRH antagonists like cetrorelix or ganirelix are used to

prevent premature ovulation during the stimulation process.
- **Triggering Ovulation:** Once the follicles reach an optimal size (typically around 15 to 18 mm), an injection of human chorionic gonadotropin (hCG) is administered to trigger ovulation. This injection is usually given in the evening, approximately 36 hours before egg retrieval. In some cases, a GnRH agonist like leuprolide may be used instead to trigger ovulation.
- **Side Effects of Treatment:** FSH injections themselves do not typically cause direct side effects. However, they lead to ovarian enlargement, which can result in abdominal swelling, discomfort, nausea, or, in severe cases, vomiting. Ovarian hyperstimulation syndrome (OHSS), characterized by extreme ovarian enlargement, can also occur. OHSS may lead to severe abdominal pain, vomiting, and, if left untreated, blood clots and fluid imbalances in the blood. Strategies to reduce OHSS risk include using GnRH agonist medication, avoiding immediate embryo transfer, or, in rare cases, cycle cancellation.
- **Egg Retrieval**: Approximately 35 to 36 hours after the hCG or leuprolide injection, a critical step in the IVF process takes place: egg retrieval. During this procedure, an ultrasound probe is inserted into the vagina, followed by a needle to gently

extract eggs from each follicle. This process typically takes between 15 to 30 minutes and is performed under conscious sedation, ensuring comfort throughout.

- **Egg Retrieval Side Effects:** Following the egg retrieval procedure, patients are monitored in a recovery area for several hours before going home. Due to the effects of anesthesia, patients should not drive or return to work for roughly 24 hours. Common side effects include pelvic cramping, light bleeding, and vaginal discharge. Any persistent or severe problems should be reported to a healthcare provider, as they might indicate early OHSS.
- **Fertilization:** The retrieved eggs are combined with sperm within a laboratory dish, allowing fertilization to occur. The sperm source can be from a partner or a donor bank. Approximately 65% of eggs are typically successfully fertilized through this process.
- **Intracytoplasmic Sperm Injection (ICSI):** In cases of severe male factor infertility, a procedure called Intracytoplasmic Sperm Injection (ICSI) is employed. This technique involves injecting a single sperm into an egg using a micro-needle and a microscope. ICSI is an option for those with severe male factor infertility, regardless of sperm count.

- **Embryo Transfer:** Embryos can be transferred fresh, a few days after egg retrieval, or after cryopreservation. The choice between fresh and frozen transfer often depends on PGT results, among other factors.
- **Fresh Embryo Transfer:** Generally performed on day three or day five after egg retrieval, this involves placing one or more embryos into the uterus using a flexible catheter.
- **Frozen Embryo Transfer:** This approach involves using embryos previously frozen and thawed. It is more common due to the additional time required for PGT results.
- **Procedure and Aftercare:** The embryo transfer procedure is typically straightforward, and anesthesia is not usually required. A speculum is placed in the vagina, and a soft plastic catheter is gently inserted through the cervix. Minimizing uterine cramping is essential for a successful transfer. Patients are often encouraged to rest at home for several hours post-transfer, although studies do not indicate that rest significantly increases the chances of pregnancy.
- **Progesterone Medication:** Most clinicians prescribe progesterone medication post-transfer to enhance embryo implantation. Progesterone can be administered in various forms, including vaginal gel, suppositories, or intramuscular injections.

- **Number of Embryos to Transfer:** The decision on how many embryos to transfer is influenced by various factors, including age, pregnancy history, embryo quality, and personal preferences. Younger individuals undergoing their first IVF cycle are typically advised to transfer only one embryo. However, if multiple IVF cycles fail to yield a pregnancy, doctors may recommend transferring more embryos, albeit at the cost of an increased risk of multiple gestations.
- **Storing Unused Embryos:** Embryos that are not transferred can be cryopreserved (frozen). The success rates for frozen and fresh embryos are similar, offering flexibility for future attempts at conception. Patients have several options for these unused embryos: they can be transferred in a subsequent cycle, donated for research or another couple's use, or disposed of.
- **PGT of Embryos:** PGT is a valuable tool that can assess the number of chromosomes (PGT-A), test for specific diseases or gene abnormalities (PGT-M) or evaluate chromosome structure (PGT-SR). PGT offers more control over the genetic health of embryos. However, it's important to note that PGT is not infallible, and standard prenatal testing is still necessary for pregnancies resulting from PGT.
- **PGT-A:** This test determines if embryos are chromosomally normal (euploid) or abnormal

(aneuploid). It is performed when embryos reach the blastocyst stage, typically between days five to seven.
- **PGT-M:** Couples with known genetic mutations may opt for PGT-M to screen embryos for specific diseases or gene abnormalities. This is especially relevant when both partners carry genes for conditions like cystic fibrosis or sickle cell anemia.
- **PGT-SR:** In rare cases of recurrent pregnancy loss due to one partner having a translocation (exchange of genetic material between two chromosomes), PGT-SR can be employed to screen embryos for these translocations.
- **Chromosomal Testing for Sex Selection:** In certain situations, embryos can undergo chromosomal testing for sex selection. This may be chosen when there is a significant risk of a gender-related disease or as part of family planning.
- **Testing's Imperfection:** It's crucial to understand that while PGT is a powerful tool, it is not foolproof, and pregnancies resulting from PGT still require standard prenatal testing. PGT is not routinely recommended for all embryos but rather is decided on an individual basis.

Testing for Pregnancy After IVF

After all the stages of IVF, the moment of truth arrives—testing for pregnancy. Two main methods are employed (Ho, 2023):

- **Blood Testing**: Approximately two weeks after the embryo transfer, a blood test for human chorionic gonadotropin (hCG) is scheduled. This hormone is a reliable indicator of pregnancy, and blood testing offers greater sensitivity than home urine pregnancy tests.
- **Home Urine Pregnancy Tests**: Home tests are not typically recommended after IVF, as they are less sensitive and may yield false-negative results, causing undue anxiety.
- **Interpreting Blood Test Results**: The initial blood hCG level measurement is crucial. A level below five international units/L indicates that pregnancy has not occurred. A level above 10 international units/L usually prompts a repeat test after 48 hours to ensure hCG levels are increasing as expected. During early pregnancy, hCG levels should roughly double every 48 hours.
- **Ultrasound**: If hCG levels progress as anticipated, a pelvic ultrasound is typically scheduled three to four weeks after the embryo transfer. This ultrasound allows healthcare providers to visualize a gestational sac within the uterus. At

around five to six weeks of pregnancy (three to four weeks after the transfer), the yolk sac becomes visible. Fetal cardiac activity, or a heartbeat, can usually be observed between 6 to 6.5 weeks of pregnancy (4 to 4.5 weeks post-transfer).

Pregnancy Care

Assuming a successful pregnancy is achieved, prenatal care becomes the next priority. Typically, prenatal care begins around six to ten weeks into the pregnancy (Ho, 2023). During this period, individuals will commence regular visits to their obstetrician, nurse, or midwife. These check-ups enable healthcare providers to monitor both the expectant parent and the developing fetus, ensuring everything progresses smoothly. It's also an opportunity to address any questions or concerns.

Predicting the Outcome of IVF

Predicting the outcome of IVF can be challenging, but predictive models have been developed to provide insight into the likelihood of success. These models consider various factors, such as age and the number of IVF cycles (Ho, 2023). By inputting specific data into these models, individuals considering IVF can obtain an estimate of their expected outcomes.

One such model is available for free on the Society for Assisted Reproductive Technology (SART) website (Ho,

2023). It provides predictions for success over the course of multiple cycles and the effect of transferring one or two embryos on live birth rates and multiple birth rates.

When IVF Is Not Successful

While IVF offers hope to many, it's essential to understand that it may not always lead to success. IVF success rates vary based on age, the cause of infertility, and treatment approaches (Ho, 2023).

For instance, data from the United States in 2021 showed that the live birth rate for each IVF cycle started was approximately (Ho, 2023):

- 45% for individuals under 35 years
- 32% for individuals aged 35 to 37
- 21% for individuals aged 38 to 40
- 10% for individuals aged 41 to 42
- 3% for individuals over 42

The success rates of individual infertility clinics can be found on the Society for Assisted Reproductive Technology (SART) website.

Coping with the emotional highs and lows of infertility treatment can be challenging. This is particularly true for those who experience unsuccessful IVF cycles. It's essential to have a strong support network, which may include partners, friends, family, or mental health professionals who specialize in fertility issues.

The Financial Aspect of IVF

IVF can be financially taxing, and it's essential to prepare for the associated costs. These costs vary widely depending on location, clinic, and individual circumstances (Ho, 2023).

- **Initial Consultation:** The initial consultation typically costs several hundred dollars and may or may not be covered by insurance.
- **Diagnostic Testing:** Diagnostic tests can range from a few hundred to several thousand dollars, depending on the extent and type of testing required.
- **Medications:** Fertility medications can cost anywhere from a few thousand to several thousand dollars per cycle. Some insurance plans may cover part of these costs.
- **IVF Cycle:** The core IVF cycle includes ovarian stimulation, egg retrieval, and embryo transfer. The average cost per IVF cycle in the United States is approximately $12,000 to $15,000, excluding medications and other ancillary services.
- **Cryopreservation:** Costs for freezing and storing embryos can vary, with annual fees ranging from a few hundred to a few thousand dollars.

- **Additional Services:** PGT, intracytoplasmic sperm injection (ICSI), and other services add to the overall cost.
- **Insurance Coverage:** Some insurance plans may cover portions of IVF treatments, while others may not cover any aspect. It's crucial to verify coverage with your insurance provider.
- **Financial Planning:** Considering the financial implications is a crucial aspect of preparing for IVF. Some individuals or couples choose to take out loans or explore financing options specifically designed for fertility treatments.

Legal and Ethical Considerations

IVF raises a range of legal and ethical considerations, which can vary by country and region. Some key issues to be aware of include (Ho, 2023):

- **Consent:** Clear and informed consent is a fundamental aspect of IVF. Individuals should fully understand the procedures, risks, and potential outcomes before embarking on treatment.
- **Disposition of Embryos:** Decisions about what to do with unused embryos can be legally complex. It's important to clarify your wishes and potentially involve legal counsel when making these decisions.

- **Donor and Surrogacy Agreements:** If you are using donor sperm, eggs, or embryos, or if you are considering gestational surrogacy, it's crucial to have legally binding agreements in place to protect the rights and responsibilities of all parties involved.
- **Ethical Concerns:** Ethical questions may arise, such as those related to selective reduction (reducing the number of embryos in the womb), sex selection, or genetic testing. Seek guidance from healthcare providers and ethicists when facing such decisions.

The Emotional Rollercoaster of IVF

The IVF journey is often an emotional rollercoaster, filled with highs and lows. It's essential to prioritize emotional well-being throughout the process. Here are some strategies (Ho, 2023):

- **Support System:** Lean on your partner, friends, and family for emotional support. Many couples find that sharing their experiences with others who have undergone IVF can be particularly helpful.
- **Counseling:** Consider seeking counseling or therapy, either individually or as a couple. Professionals with expertise in fertility and

reproductive health can provide valuable guidance.
- **Self-Care:** Prioritize self-care activities that reduce stress, such as yoga, meditation, or simply spending time doing things you enjoy.
- **Expect the Unexpected:** Understand that IVF can be unpredictable. Not all cycles will result in pregnancy, and there may be setbacks along the way. Be prepared for unexpected outcomes and setbacks and allow yourself to grieve and heal as needed.
- **Communication:** Maintain open and honest communication with your healthcare team. They can provide valuable insights, answer questions, and help you make informed decisions.

Embarking on the IVF journey is a significant decision that can bring hope and joy to those facing fertility challenges. It's a complex process that involves numerous steps, medical interventions, and emotional ups and downs. Understanding what IVF entails, who it's suitable for, and the potential outcomes and challenges is essential for anyone considering this path to parenthood.

While IVF can be a life-changing experience, it's vital to approach it with realistic expectations and a strong support system. The emotional, physical, and financial demands can be significant. Still, with the right guidance and a resilient spirit, many individuals and couples achieve their dreams of building a family through IVF (Ho, 2023). Remember that no matter the outcome, your worth and love as an individual or couple extend far beyond your ability to conceive, and there are many paths to a fulfilling and meaningful life.

INTRAUTERINE INSEMINATION (IUI)

If you're on the exhilarating journey to parenthood but have hit some bumps in the road, fear not. There's a fertility superhero in town, and its name is intrauterine insemination, or IUI for short.

In this section, we're going to delve deep into the world of IUI, breaking down the important details.

The Lowdown on IUI: What's It All About?

To kick things off, let's understand the basics. IUI, also known as artificial insemination, is a fertility procedure designed to give sperm a helping hand in reaching its destination—the uterus (Mayo Clinic, 2019). Its primary goal is to increase the chances of sperm fertilizing an egg, ultimately leading to pregnancy.

Perfect Timing is Key

One of the crucial elements of IUI is perfect timing. This isn't a game of chance; it's about orchestrating a meeting between sperm and egg with precision. This rendezvous typically occurs around the time when your ovaries are about to release an egg or two during ovulation. Picture it as setting up a romantic encounter in the fallopian tube, where the sperm and egg can unite and work their magic to create a baby (Mayo Clinic, 2019).

Why Choose IUI?

Now, let's explore why someone might opt for IUI as their go-to fertility solution (Mayo Clinic, 2019):

- **Donor Sperm:** If you're flying solo, your partner doesn't have viable sperm, or their sperm quality is less than stellar, donor sperm can be your knight in shining armor. IUI ensures that these superhero sperm have a clear path to success. Donor sperm is carefully selected, obtained from certified labs, and thawed before the IUI procedure.
- **Unexplained Infertility:** Sometimes, Mother Nature keeps her secrets hidden, leaving couples baffled about their infertility. In such cases, IUI is often the first step in the journey to parenthood. Fertility medications might also join the party to enhance your chances of conceiving.
- **Endometriosis-Related Infertility:** Endometriosis is a pesky condition where tissue similar to the uterine lining grows outside the uterus. It can wreak havoc on your fertility plans. Typically, the initial approach to tackle endometriosis-related infertility involves using

medications to prepare your body for a successful egg release, coupled with IUI.
- **Mild Male Factor Infertility (Subfertility):** Sometimes, the roadblock to pregnancy lies in the quality or quantity of sperm. A semen analysis, which examines sperm quantity, size, shape, and motility, helps diagnose these issues (Mayo Clinic, 2019). IUI can be a game-changer in such scenarios. By preparing the sperm for the procedure, it becomes possible to select the highest-quality sperm, giving them a VIP ticket to the uterus.
- **Cervical Factor Infertility:** Problems with the cervix can be a roadblock to conception. The cervix, which acts as the gateway between the vagina and uterus, produces mucus during ovulation to help sperm reach the egg. If this mucus is too thick or the cervix itself is causing issues, IUI can sidestep these obstacles by directly placing sperm into the uterus. Additionally, scarring from procedures like biopsies can thicken the cervix, making IUI a valuable workaround.
- **Ovulatory Factor Infertility:** IUI is a viable option for individuals dealing with infertility due to ovulation problems. This category includes cases where there's either a lack of ovulation or a reduced number of eggs being released during the menstrual cycle. Fertility medications often

complement IUI to ensure ovulation occurs at the right time.
- **Semen Allergy:** Yes, it's rare, but some individuals are allergic to proteins in semen. When semen comes into contact with the skin, it can cause painful reactions like burning and swelling. Condoms can provide relief but also prevent pregnancy. IUI comes to the rescue by removing many of the allergenic proteins from the sperm before insemination. This allows for pregnancy while avoiding the unpleasant symptoms associated with the allergy.

What About the Risks?

Every superhero has its Kryptonite, and IUI is no exception. However, the risks associated with IUI are generally minimal. Nevertheless, it is important to go in with your eyes open to every possibility (Mayo Clinic, 2019).

- **Infection:** There's a slight chance of infection following an IUI procedure. Rest assured, though—this is a rare occurrence.
- **Spotting:** During IUI, a catheter is gently placed through the vagina and into the uterus to deliver the sperm. Occasionally, this process can lead to minimal vaginal bleeding, often referred to as spotting. It's typically nothing to be concerned about and rarely affects the chances of pregnancy.

- **Multiple Pregnancy:** IUI itself doesn't inherently increase the likelihood of having twins, triplets, or more. However, when fertility medications are combined with IUI, the chances of multiple pregnancies do rise. Multiple pregnancies carry higher risks compared to single pregnancies, such as premature labor and low birth weight, so it's essential to consider this when deciding on your fertility treatment plan.

Preparing for the Big Day

Alright, you're on board with IUI—what's next? In the build-up to IUI, there are a few things you will have to do for the actual process (Mayo Clinic, 2019):

- **Ovulation Monitoring:** Given that timing is of the essence in IUI, monitoring your ovulation is crucial. You can achieve this using an at-home ovulation predictor kit (OPK), which detects the surge of LH responsible for triggering ovulation. Alternatively, your healthcare provider might perform a transvaginal ultrasound to visualize your ovaries and monitor egg development. In some cases, you might receive an injection of human chorionic gonadotropin (HCG) or other medications to ensure your eggs are ready for action at the right moment.

- **Perfect Timing:** Your healthcare provider will create a carefully choreographed plan that specifies the ideal timing for your IUI procedure. This ensures that sperm and egg have the best chance of encountering each other in the right place at the right time.
- **Sperm Preparation:** Now, it's time to prepare the star of the show – the sperm. If you're using your partner's sperm, they'll need to provide a sample at the doctor's office. Don't worry; it's a breeze. The sample is processed to separate the cream of the crop, the high-quality sperm, from the rest. This process also eliminates any elements that could cause adverse reactions, such as severe cramps, if introduced into the uterus. The idea is to maximize your chances of pregnancy by using a small, highly concentrated sample of healthy sperm.

The IUI Showdown: What to Expect During the Procedure

Here comes the big moment—the IUI procedure itself (Mayo Clinic, 2019). Visualize it as the climax of your fertility journey, where the magic unfolds:

- **Setting the Stage:** You'll find yourself in a comfortable examination room, your legs placed in stirrups (not the most glamorous pose, we

admit). Your trusted healthcare provider, be it your doctor or a skilled nurse, takes the stage.
- **Sperm Delivery:** The procedure kicks off with precision. A tiny tube, known as a catheter, is attached to a vial containing the meticulously prepared sperm – the cream of the crop. The catheter is gently guided through the cervix and into the uterus, where the sperm are released with the utmost care.
- **The Grand Finale:** Once the sperm has been placed within your uterus, the catheter and speculum are removed. And just like that, you've completed your IUI procedure. It's all done in a matter of minutes, and you'll likely feel minimal to no discomfort.

After the Show: Recovery and What to Expect

After the IUI extravaganza, you're not in for an extended recovery period. Here's what you can anticipate (Mayo Clinic, 2019):

- **Light Spotting:** You might experience some light spotting for a day or two after the procedure. This is entirely normal and should not be cause for concern. It's usually a minor inconvenience at most.
- **Return to Normal:** Following the procedure, you can go about your daily routine without any

significant interruptions. There is no need for bed rest or special precautions—life goes on as usual.

The Waiting Game: Pregnancy Testing

Now, the patience game begins. You've done your part, and the sperm are on their mission. It's time to give them the space they need to work their magic. You should wait for approximately two weeks before taking an at-home pregnancy test.

Beware of Testing Too Early

This is the part where many aspiring parents find it tough to resist the urge to test prematurely. However, it's crucial to exercise patience and not jump the gun. Testing too soon can lead to misleading results (Mayo Clinic, 2019):

- **False-Negative:** Testing too early might yield a "no pregnancy" result when you're, in fact, pregnant. This occurs because it takes time for pregnancy hormones to reach detectable levels.
- **False-Positive:** On the flip side, testing too early can result in a "pregnant" result when you're not actually pregnant. This can happen if you've recently taken fertility medications like HCG, which can linger in your system and produce a false-positive result.

What If It Doesn't Work?

Now, let's address the scenario where the test results aren't the joyful news you were hoping for. Remember, it's okay—these things can take time. If you don't achieve pregnancy with your first IUI attempt, don't lose hope. Many individuals undergo multiple rounds of IUI, often between three to six cycles, to maximize their chances of success.

There you have it—the ins and outs of IUI, your trusty sidekick on the path to parenthood. It's essential to approach this journey with optimism and patience. While IUI can work wonders for many, it may take time and several attempts to reach your goal of becoming a parent (Mayo Clinic, 2019).

Remember, every step you take brings you one step closer to realizing your dream of a family. So, embrace the process, stay positive, and trust that your superhero, IUI, is doing its utmost to make your dreams of parenthood a reality.

THE EMOTIONAL JOURNEY OF FERTILITY TREATMENTS

If you've ever been on a roller coaster, you're probably familiar with the rush of emotions that accompany the twists, turns, and unpredictable ups and downs. Well, the emotional journey of fertility treatment is a lot like that roller coaster, complete with its highs and lows, moments of exhilaration, and times of heartache and uncertainty. It's a ride that's deeply personal and profoundly emotional, and it's crucial to acknowledge and validate the range of emotions that individuals and couples experience throughout this transformative process (*Emotional and Psychological Aspects of Fertility Treatment*, 2023).

The Roller Coaster of Emotions

The fertility treatment journey often begins with a spark of hope and excitement. You've made the decision to pursue your dreams of parenthood, and that initial step is filled with anticipation and optimism. But as you progress through the process, you may encounter obstacles, setbacks, and moments of disappointment. These emotional lows can be challenging, leaving you feeling frustrated, discouraged, and even heartbroken.

Anxiety becomes a constant companion as you navigate the uncertainties and unknowns of fertility treatment. Each step of the way brings new questions and anxieties: Will this cycle be successful? What if it's not? How do we cope with the emotional toll of another negative result? Understanding and acknowledging this emotional roller coaster is vital both for individuals and couples. It's about giving yourself permission to feel, to express your emotions, and to seek strategies for effectively managing them.

Relationship Challenges on the Journey

Fertility treatment doesn't just affect individuals; it also places significant strain on relationships. Couples, in particular, may encounter unique challenges as they navigate the complexities of fertility treatment together. The stress and pressure of the process can lead to communication breakdowns and strains on even the strongest bonds. Furthermore, the emotional ups and downs experienced by each partner can further complicate matters.

However, it's essential to recognize that fertility treatment has the potential to bring couples closer together. It can foster resilience, mutual support, and a deeper understanding of one another. Open and honest communication is key, allowing both partners to express their fears, frustrations, and hopes. Quality time together, devoid of fertility-related discussions, can help maintain a sense of connection and intimacy (*Emotional and Psychological Aspects of Fertility Treatment,* 2023). And when needed, seeking professional guidance from therapists or counselors can provide invaluable tools for navigating relationship challenges successfully.

Coping With Uncertainty and Loss

Uncertainty and loss are inherent aspects of fertility treatment, and they can take a profound emotional toll. Coping with the uncertainty of whether each treatment cycle will be successful can be incredibly challenging (*Emotional and Psychological Aspects of Fertility Treatment,*

2023). Individuals and couples may grapple with a range of emotions, including fear, anxiety, and sadness. Moreover, the experience of pregnancy loss or unsuccessful treatment cycles can bring about profound grief and feelings of loss.

Navigating the Uncertainty

To navigate the uncertainty of fertility treatments, it's essential to focus on self-care and stress management. Engaging in activities that promote relaxation, such as yoga, meditation, or journaling, can provide a sense of calm and stability amidst the turbulence. Setting realistic expectations and cultivating patience can help individuals cope with the ever-present uncertainty of the treatment process (*Emotional and Psychological Aspects of Fertility Treatment*, 2023). Seeking support from loved ones, participating in support groups, or consulting with mental health professionals can offer guidance and comfort.

Coping With Loss

Experiencing pregnancy loss or unsuccessful treatment cycles can be devastating. It's essential to acknowledge and honor the grief associated with these losses. Allowing yourself to grieve and express your emotions freely is a vital part of the healing process. Seeking support from others who have gone through similar experiences, whether through support groups or online communities, can offer a sense of understanding and solace.

Engaging in self-compassion and self-care practices can be transformative during the grieving process (*Emotional and Psychological Aspects of Fertility Treatment*, 2023). Pursuing hobbies, seeking therapy, or finding healthy emotional outlets can help individuals navigate the challenging journey of coping with loss.

Seeking Support and Building Resilience

Amid this emotional roller coaster, support and resilience play critical roles in maintaining emotional well-being. Building a robust support network and accessing professional help can provide individuals and couples with the tools they need to navigate their challenges successfully (*Emotional and Psychological Aspects of Fertility Treatment*, 2023). Additionally, cultivating resilience can help individuals bounce back from setbacks and maintain a positive outlook.

The Importance of Support Networks

Creating a support network of understanding family members, friends, or support groups can provide a safe space to share experiences, emotions, and concerns. Connecting with others who have gone through or are currently undergoing fertility treatment can offer a sense of validation, empathy, and encouragement (*Emotional and Psychological Aspects of Fertility Treatment*, 2023). Online forums and social media platforms dedicated to fertility can also serve as valuable sources of support and information.

Seeking Professional Help

In some cases, professional help from therapists, counselors, or psychologists can be incredibly beneficial. These professionals can provide specialized guidance and support tailored to the emotional and psychological challenges of fertility treatment. Therapy sessions offer individuals and couples a dedicated space to explore their feelings, learn effective coping strategies, and strengthen their mental and emotional well-being (*Emotional and Psychological Aspects of Fertility Treatment*, 2023).

Building Resilience

Building resilience is a cornerstone of navigating the ups and downs of fertility treatment. Practicing self-care, engaging in stress-reducing activities, and maintaining a healthy lifestyle can contribute to overall well-being. Taking breaks when needed, pursuing hobbies that bring joy, and prioritizing self-compassion can help individuals stay grounded and resilient during difficult moments (*Emotional and Psychological Aspects of Fertility Treatment*, 2023). Developing a positive mindset, reframing negative thoughts, and setting realistic expectations can also build resilience on this journey.

Fertility treatment is not just a medical process; it's a deeply personal and emotionally charged journey. By prioritizing emotional well-being alongside the medical aspects, we create a more supportive environment for those on this transformative path. Let's provide understanding, empathy, and guidance to empower individuals and couples as they pursue their dreams of parenthood (*Emotional and Psychological Aspects of Fertility Treatment*, 2023). Remember, you're not alone on this roller coaster—there's a supportive community ready to stand by your side, offering strength and hope as you navigate the twists and turns of fertility treatment.

Body, Mind, Heart—Go All-in!

In the world of fertility treatment, resilience is the unsung hero, the quiet strength that allows individuals and couples to persevere through the unpredictable twists and turns of this deeply personal journey. It's the unwavering determination to hold onto hope even in the face of setbacks, the courage to face uncertainty head-on, and the capacity to heal and grow after experiencing loss.

Along this path, it's important to remember that sometimes, despite your best efforts and the unwavering support you receive, losses may still occur. These moments of heartbreak and grief are an integral part of the journey, but they don't define your entire story. They are the shadows that make the light of hope shine even brighter.

As you continue to navigate the emotional roller coaster of fertility treatment, know that you are not alone. Your resilience, your capacity to love, and your dreams of parenthood are the driving forces that will carry you forward. Reach out to your support network, seek professional guidance when needed, and embrace the strength within you.

The path to parenthood may be challenging, but it is also a testament to the remarkable resilience of the human spirit. Your journey is unique, and your strength is unparalleled. Keep moving forward, for hope persists, and your dreams are worth every step.

WHISPERS OF STRENGTH— HEALING AND HOPE AFTER PREGNANCY LOSS

LAURA AND BEX'S PATHS INTERSECT

"My journey into motherhood has been a heart-wrenching odyssey, filled with trials and tribulations that have tested my spirit in ways I never imagined. Now, at 37, I carry the heavy weight of seven miscarriages, each one a poignant reminder of my fervent desire to hold my own child in my arms. With each loss, hope seemed to slip through my fingers like grains of sand, and I couldn't help but withdraw into a cocoon of despair.

As the miscarriages continued to haunt me, my longing for motherhood intensified, transcending the sorrow of losing each individual baby. It became a profound ache, an insatiable yearning that left me feeling adrift in a sea of dashed dreams.

Desperate for answers and a glimmer of hope, I embarked on a quest to seek out specialists who could unravel the enigma of my recurrent miscarriages. Finally, after a long and arduous search, I found a doctor who would become my beacon of light in the darkest of times. The diagnosis was both a revelation and a bittersweet truth—an autoimmune disease was the culprit, my own body unwittingly attacking my pregnancies.

With newfound determination and resilience, I faced my next pregnancy armed with immunosuppressants. Yet, even as the pregnancy progressed, I dared not believe it was real. The fear of another heartbreak loomed large, and I cautiously spoke of "if" the baby arrived, not "when." It was as if I had constructed an emotional fortress around myself to shield me from the pain of potential loss.

The day of my cesarean section arrived, and I, still grappling with disbelief, couldn't fathom the idea of holding a living, breathing infant in my arms. It was a moment I had yearned for, but one that had eluded me for so long.

Contrary to my fears, the bond between mother and child blossomed beautifully. My son, a testament to my unwavering determination, was not just a wonderful baby but grew into a remarkable toddler. I felt a profound sense of luck and gratitude that touched the depths of my soul.

It was during this time that I crossed paths with Bex through the vast expanse of social media. We shared a common understanding of the trials and tribulations of baby loss and pregnancy after miscarriage. Both of us believed that more needed to be done to support others on this emotionally turbulent journey.

Together, we embarked on a mission to create a haven of support and understanding. Thus, "The Worst Girl Gang Ever" was born—a podcast, a support group, a learning platform, and a book, all aimed at helping women navigate the labyrinth of life after baby loss. Bex and I wanted to shatter the silence surrounding the struggles of motherhood and create a safe space where women could share their stories and find solace in the company of those who understood.

Bex aptly pointed out the absence of a narrative where motherhood doesn't follow the expected script, where the journey is marred by loss and uncertainty. We aimed to change that by bringing these hidden stories into the light, empowering women to embrace their unique paths to motherhood.

In the end, my story is a testament to the resilience of the human spirit. It's a reminder that even in the darkest of times, hope can flicker to life, and dreams can be realized. My journey, though fraught with pain and sorrow, ultimately led me to a place of profound joy and gratitude, proving that the most arduous paths can lead to the most beautiful destinations" (*Pregnancy After Miscarriage*, n.d.).

MISCARRIAGES AND PREGNANCY LOSS

Miscarriage, often referred to as early pregnancy loss, is a journey through heartbreak that touches the lives of countless women. It's a profound loss that occurs before the 20-week mark of pregnancy. For those who recognize their pregnancies, statistics tell us that roughly 10 to 20 in every 100 pregnancies, or 10-20%, end in miscarriage (*Miscarriage*, 2023). It's an agonizing reality that many must face, but it's essential to remember that you are not alone, and support is available.

The Timing of Loss

Timing plays a significant role in the experience of miscarriage. The majority, approximately 80%, occur within the first trimester, before the 12th week of pregnancy (*Miscarriage*, 2023). The first trimester is a period of profound vulnerability, where hopes and dreams of the future often hang by a thread.

In the second trimester, from weeks 13 to 19, the occurrence of miscarriage decreases, but it's not entirely absent. Roughly one in five in every 100 pregnancies, or one to five percent, may experience this heart-wrenching loss during this time. Beyond the 20-week mark, when pregnancy loss occurs, it's termed as stillbirth, another devastating chapter in the realm of pregnancy-related grief (*Miscarriage*, 2023).

Different Forms of Miscarriage

- **Threatened Miscarriage:** This term applies when a pregnant person experiences bleeding, minimal or no pain, and a cervix that remains closed (undilated). In some cases, the heartbeat of the baby can still be detected. Fortunately, most threatened miscarriages resolve without further complications (*Miscarriage*, 2023).
- **Incomplete Miscarriage:** When a miscarriage begins, but the body doesn't expel all the pregnancy tissue, it is considered incomplete. Symptoms may include bleeding, cramping, and signs of miscarriage (*Miscarriage*, 2023).
- **Complete Miscarriage:** In contrast, a complete miscarriage signifies that the body has successfully expelled all pregnancy tissue. Sometimes, this process happens suddenly, or it may require medical intervention (*Miscarriage*, 2023).
- **Asymptomatic Miscarriage:** This form of miscarriage is particularly perplexing as it occurs without the typical signs of bleeding or cramping. Individuals may not even pass any tissue from their body. In some cases, this is referred to as an empty sac pregnancy, and a medical procedure may be necessary to remove the pregnancy tissue (*Miscarriage*, 2023).

Recurrent Pregnancy Loss: A Heartbreaking Journey

For a small but significant group of individuals, miscarriage isn't a singular event but a recurring nightmare. This condition, known as recurrent pregnancy loss or repeat miscarriages, is defined by the loss of two pregnancies in succession. Approximately 1 in 100 pregnant people, or one percent, face this heart-wrenching challenge (Miscarriage, 2023).

The emotional toll of experiencing a second miscarriage is staggering. It's estimated that after two consecutive miscarriages, the risk of yet another heartbreaking loss increases to about 28 in 100 or 28%. And for those who endure three or more miscarriages in succession, the risk of facing another miscarriage climbs to a daunting 43 in 100 or 43% (Miscarriage, 2023).

Unraveling the Mysteries of Miscarriage

While we may never fully understand the causes of every miscarriage, some factors are known to contribute to these heartbreaking losses. One of the most common culprits is chromosomal abnormalities, responsible for up to seven in every ten, or 70%, of all miscarriages (*Miscarriage*, 2023). These abnormalities usually occur randomly and are not typically inherited.

Chromosomes, the structures within our cells that contain genes, come in pairs, with each person inheriting one chromosome from each parent. Miscarriages that occur within the first three months of pregnancy often result from chromosomal issues. Examples include conditions such as a blighted ovum, where an embryo doesn't develop, and intrauterine fetal demise, where an embryo stops growing (*Miscarriage*, 2023).

Translocation, a condition where part of a chromosome moves to another, accounts for a smaller percentage of repeat miscarriages. Additionally, other chromosome issues like anencephaly, trisomies, renal agenesis, and hydrops can also contribute to pregnancy loss (*Miscarriage*, 2023).

Beyond Chromosomes: Other Factors

While chromosomal abnormalities are a common factor, they aren't the sole contributors to miscarriage. Problems within the uterus or cervix can also play a role. Conditions like a septate uterus, Asherman syndrome, fibroids, polyps, or cervical insufficiency can lead to miscarriages between the 12th and 20th weeks of pregnancy (*Miscarriage*, 2023).

Infections, too, can have dire consequences for a pregnancy. Some infections like Parvovirus B19, cytomegalovirus, sexually transmitted infections (STIs), and listeriosis have the potential to cause miscarriage (*Miscarriage*, 2023). Early detection and treatment of infections are vital for protecting both the pregnant person and their baby.

Facing the Unknown

Miscarriage is a deeply personal and often bewildering journey. While we strive to unravel its mysteries and minimize its occurrence, one thing is certain: support is essential. Whether you are confronting a single miscarriage, the challenges of recurrent pregnancy loss, or facing the complexities of pregnancy after loss, remember that you are not alone.

Seek comfort in the knowledge that countless others have walked this path before you and emerged stronger. Support organizations like Share Pregnancy and Infant Loss Support in the United States and Tommy's in the United Kingdom are dedicated to providing guidance, understanding, and a sense of community (*Miscarriage*, 2023).

Though the road may be treacherous and uncertain, it's vital to remember that most people who experience miscarriages go on to have healthy pregnancies later. Hold on to hope, lean on your support system, and, most importantly, be kind to yourself. In the face of miscarriage, resilience often emerges as a beacon of light, guiding you toward brighter days.

Assessing Your Risk

It's essential to be aware of specific risk factors that might increase the likelihood of miscarriage (*Miscarriage*, 2023):

- **Previous Miscarriages:** Having experienced two or more previous miscarriages can raise your risk, underscoring the importance of seeking appropriate medical guidance and support.
- **Age:** As age advances, particularly for those aged 35 and older, the risk of miscarriage increases. Importantly, the age of the partner can also influence this risk.
- **Substance Use:** Smoking, consuming alcohol, or using street drugs like cocaine or methamphetamines during pregnancy can heighten the risk of miscarriage. Seeking help to quit is essential for a healthier pregnancy.
- **Exposure to Harmful Chemicals:** Contact with harmful chemicals such as solvents, which dissolve substances like certain detergent mixtures and paint thinner, can elevate the risk of miscarriage (*Miscarriage*, 2023). Exposure to substances like lead, arsenic, radiation, or air pollution also poses potential dangers. Consult with your healthcare provider to determine how best to protect yourself and your baby from such risks.

Health Conditions and Miscarriage

Certain health conditions can increase the risk of miscarriage (*Miscarriage*, 2023). Early identification and proper management of these conditions are crucial:

- **Autoimmune Disorders:** These conditions, where the body mistakenly attacks its healthy tissues, can elevate the risk of miscarriage. Antiphospholipid syndrome and lupus (systemic lupus erythematosus or SLE) are among the autoimmune disorders associated with an increased risk. Individuals with antiphospholipid syndrome and a history of recurrent miscarriages may receive low-dose aspirin and heparin during pregnancy to reduce the risk.
- **Obesity:** A BMI of 30 or higher indicates obesity and can contribute to an increased risk of miscarriage. Prior to pregnancy, addressing obesity through healthy lifestyle changes can be beneficial.
- **Hormone Problems:** Conditions like PCOS and luteal phase defect, characterized by low levels of progesterone over multiple menstrual cycles, can be associated with miscarriage. Treatment with progesterone before and during pregnancy may be recommended to mitigate the risk.
- **Preexisting Health Conditions:** Conditions like diabetes, hypertension, thyroid disorders, severe kidney disease, congenital heart disease, and severe malnutrition may heighten the risk of miscarriage. Careful management and monitoring before and during pregnancy are crucial in these cases.

- **Group B Strep Infection:** This infection can be associated with an increased risk of miscarriage. Timely detection and appropriate medical intervention are essential for protecting both the pregnant person and their baby.

Other Factors and Their Influence

Several additional factors can also impact the risk of miscarriage (*Miscarriage*, 2023):

- **Certain Medications:** Some studies suggest that nonsteroidal anti-inflammatory medications (NSAIDs), such as ibuprofen, naproxen, and diclofenac, might increase the risk of miscarriage. The acne medication isotretinoin has also been linked to miscarriage and fetal abnormalities.
- **Intrauterine Device (IUD) Use:** While rare, some individuals may become pregnant while using an IUD.
- **Stress:** Both intense short-term stress and chronic long-term stress can potentially elevate the risk of miscarriage. It's essential to manage stress levels and seek support when needed.
- **Social Determinants of Health:** Factors like racial, ethnic, or financial inequalities, exposure to violence, homelessness, or food insecurity can negatively affect overall health and increase the risk of miscarriage.

Understanding Caffeine and Physical Activity

While the effect of caffeine on pregnancy requires further research, it's advisable to limit daily caffeine intake to 200 milligrams (*Miscarriage*, 2023). This is approximately the amount found in a 12-ounce cup of coffee. As for physical activity and sexual activity during pregnancy, there is no evidence to support claims that they cause miscarriage.

Preventing Miscarriage

While miscarriages typically cannot be prevented, prioritizing pre-pregnancy health can reduce the risk of complications during pregnancy. This involves receiving a pre-pregnancy checkup and discussing any existing health conditions with your healthcare provider. Additionally, taking folic acid to prevent birth defects and making necessary lifestyle changes can contribute to a healthier pregnancy (*Miscarriage*, 2023).

Recognizing the Signs and Symptoms

Early recognition of the signs and symptoms of miscarriage is crucial (*Miscarriage*, 2023):

- **Bleeding:** Vaginal bleeding or spotting can be an early sign of miscarriage. While spotting is common in early pregnancy, it's essential to consult your provider if you experience any bleeding.

- **Cramps:** Cramping, similar to menstrual cramps, can be indicative of miscarriage.
- **Severe Belly Pain:** Intense abdominal pain should not be ignored and should prompt immediate medical attention.
- **Changes in Pregnancy Symptoms:** A sudden reduction in pregnancy symptoms such as nausea, breast tenderness, or fetal movement should be discussed with your provider.
- **Back Pain:** Persistent back pain may signal a problem and should be evaluated.
- **Vaginal Discharge:** Unusual vaginal discharge with a foul odor should be addressed.
- **Fever:** Developing a fever during pregnancy should be reported promptly.

Recovery and Emotional Healing

Recovery from a miscarriage can vary from person to person, typically taking several weeks to a month or longer. Pregnancy hormones may remain in the bloodstream for one to two months post-miscarriage (*Miscarriage*, 2023). Most women experience their first period again within four to six weeks.

Emotional healing often takes more time. Grieving is a personal process, and it's perfectly normal to feel sadness, anger, confusion, or isolation. Seek support from friends, family, or support groups. Find meaningful ways to remember your baby, such as preserving baby items like clothes and blankets in a special place. Remember, there is no prescribed timeline for healing; take the time you need.

Moving Forward

Deciding when to try for another pregnancy is a deeply personal choice, one to be made in consultation with your partner and healthcare provider. In many cases, it's considered safe to attempt pregnancy again after at least one normal menstrual cycle. Some studies suggest that trying soon after a miscarriage might increase the chances of conception (*Miscarriage*, 2023). Regardless of your decision, maintaining good health and taking a folic acid supplement is advisable, even if pregnancy isn't immediate.

Remember, the emotional toll of miscarriage can be profound, and it's entirely acceptable to wait before trying again. There's no rush in healing and preparing for the future. Take the time that feels right for you.

EMOTIONAL HEALING AND SUPPORT AFTER LOSS

Experiencing a miscarriage is an emotionally taxing journey, one that is often marked by a roller coaster of feelings and reactions. Whether you are the one who carried the pregnancy or you are the partner, coping with the aftermath of a miscarriage is a deeply personal and challenging experience. It's essential to understand that there is no prescribed way to feel, and the emotions you encounter are entirely valid and unique to your situation (*Your Feelings and Emotions After Miscarriage*, 2019). This section explores the complex emotions that often accompany miscarriage and offers strategies for coping and healing.

Grief: Navigating the Depths of Loss

Grief is perhaps the most profound and persistent emotion that arises after a miscarriage. It is crucial to recognize that the depth of your grief is not determined by how far along you were in your pregnancy. Even if you did not have the opportunity to meet or hold your baby, your grief is legitimate. Many women and couples begin forming a profound bond with their unborn child from the moment they discover the pregnancy (*Your Feelings and Emotions After Miscarriage*, 2019). When that connection is suddenly severed, the loss can be overwhelming.

The grief experienced after a miscarriage is not limited to the loss of a pregnancy; it extends to the dreams and hopes you had for your baby. These dreams often begin the moment you learn that you are expecting. Allow yourself to mourn not only the tangible loss but also the intangible future you had envisioned with your child.

Sarah's story serves as a poignant example (*Your Feelings and Emotions After Miscarriage*, 2019):

"I am a mother of three—the unusual bit is that our three are not with us... I'd had hope and dreams for all my little ones, I'd loved them fiercely and wanted to protect them."

Shock: The Unexpected Unfolds

Miscarriage can strike suddenly and without warning, leaving individuals and couples in a state of profound shock. This sense of bewilderment is entirely normal, regardless of whether the miscarriage was anticipated or not. Some women may even discover the loss during a routine medical appointment for an ultrasound scan, a situation referred to as a "missed miscarriage" (*Your Feelings and Emotions After Miscarriage*, 2019).

In these moments of shock, it can be challenging to make sense of what has happened. The abruptness of a miscarriage can leave individuals grappling with an overwhelming sense of disbelief and denial.

Marta's experience exemplifies this (*Your Feelings and Emotions After Miscarriage*, 2019):

"One minute, we were sitting happy and excited in the waiting room, ready to see our baby for the first time. The next we were being ushered to a different unit in the hospital to discuss how to have our baby removed. Shock doesn't begin to describe it. I hadn't had any indication there was anything wrong. I'd never even heard of a missed miscarriage. It didn't feel real."

Failure and Guilt: The Weight of Self-Blame

After a miscarriage, many individuals, particularly mothers, grapple with feelings of failure and guilt. The notion that a baby in your care, within your body, could stop growing can be profoundly distressing. You might find yourself tormented by guilt, convinced that you are somehow responsible for your baby not being born. You may question every decision, every action, and every moment leading up to the miscarriage, wondering if there was something you did or didn't do that caused your baby's brief life to end (*Your Feelings and Emotions After Miscarriage*, 2019).

It is paramount to comprehend that miscarriages very rarely occur due to something you did or did not do. The most common cause of early miscarriage, which accounts for the majority of miscarriages, is chromosomal abnormalities in the baby (*Your Feelings and Emotions After Miscarriage*, 2019). These abnormalities happen purely by chance, and no amount of care or precaution could have prevented them.

Catherine's story eloquently captures this internal struggle (*Your Feelings and Emotions After Miscarriage*, 2019):

"What if there is something I can do next time to tip the odds in my baby's favor? Because right now, if someone with a medical qualification told me I had to spend my entire pregnancy hopping on one foot while only eating broccoli and wholemeal bread, I'd do it if I thought it would raise my chances of giving birth to another healthy baby."

Emptiness: The Void Left Behind

Pregnancy often bestows a new identity upon individuals —that of a mother or parent. This identity can feel profound and transformative, making the subsequent loss all the more challenging. Many women describe a sense of emptiness following a miscarriage, a void that can be difficult to fill.

Partners may also experience this loss of identity as a parent, contributing to the complex emotional landscape. The transition from joyful anticipation to sudden emptiness can be emotionally disorienting (*Your Feelings and Emotions After Miscarriage*, 2019).

Louise's experience beautifully encapsulates this transformation: "When you get that positive pregnancy test, you are a mother-to-be. Whether it's five, 10, or 26 weeks, you are changed" (*Your Feelings and Emotions After Miscarriage*, 2019).

Loss of Control: Grappling With the Unpredictable

One of the most overwhelming aspects of parenthood, even from its earliest stages, is the realization that so much is beyond your control. You cannot dictate precisely when you get pregnant, nor can you guarantee that every pregnancy will result in a healthy baby. Instead, all you can do is follow medical advice, care for your body, and hope for the best (*Your Feelings and Emotions After Miscarriage*, 2019). For many, accepting this loss of control can be deeply challenging.

Most couples never receive a definitive explanation for why a miscarriage occurred. The absence of answers can intensify feelings of helplessness and despair.

Leanne's sentiments capture this heartbreaking uncertainty (*Your Feelings and Emotions After Miscarriage*, 2019):

"The worst part for me is the not knowing why. Why did my babies die? How could I carry a perfectly healthy child the first time and not the second or third? Why can't they test me to find out? Why? Why? Why?"

Fear: Navigating Anxiety About the Future

After experiencing a miscarriage, it is common to be consumed by fear and anxiety about future pregnancies. This fear can be all-encompassing, particularly if the cause of the miscarriage remains unknown or if it is not the first time such a loss has occurred (*Your Feelings and Emotions After Miscarriage*, 2019). Anxiety about the possibility of another miscarriage or other complications in subsequent pregnancies can be paralyzing.

These anxieties may intensify when you become pregnant again. It is essential to reach out to someone you trust and share your fears and anxieties, as opening up can alleviate some of the emotional burden (*Your Feelings and Emotions After Miscarriage*, 2019).

Jealousy: Coping with Complex Emotions Toward Others

Jealousy is a complex emotion that may rear its head after a miscarriage. You might find it challenging to feel happy for others when they announce their pregnancies or the birth of their babies. This feeling can be particularly difficult if their joyful news coincides with significant dates related to your loss. It is crucial not to judge yourself harshly for these emotions; many women who have experienced miscarriages can empathize with your feelings (*Your Feelings and Emotions After Miscarriage*, 2019).

One individual shares her experience (*Your Feelings and Emotions After Miscarriage*, 2019):

"But it just hits you from nowhere. I walked into a toilet last week in a restaurant, smack bang into a pregnant lady. It almost ruined my day. I see friends get pregnant and I resent them."

Loss of Trust in Your Body: A Disconnect Between Mind and Body

After a miscarriage, you might feel a profound disconnect between your mind and body. This sense of betrayal can be particularly potent if you experience a missed miscarriage with no physical symptoms (*Your Feelings and Emotions After Miscarriage*, 2019). You may begin to question your body's ability to carry a pregnancy to term, even in future pregnancies.

It is essential to remember that a miscarriage can affect you physically and emotionally. Your body undergoes rapid hormonal changes following a miscarriage, which can lead to mood swings and tears (*Your Feelings and Emotions After Miscarriage*, 2019). It may take time before your body and mind feel normal again.

Melissa's experience articulates this loss of trust (*Your Feelings and Emotions After Miscarriage*, 2019):

"The trouble with miscarriage is that most people don't understand what it is you've actually lost. I've lost my babies. I've lost the ability to be excited about pregnancy. I've lost trust in my body, in hospitals, and in statistics. Most of all, I've lost faith, in myself and in the future."

Confusion: Mixed Emotions and Unexpected Relief

If your pregnancy was unplanned or if you had mixed feelings about it, you might find yourself wrestling with conflicting emotions after a miscarriage. On one hand, you may have been unsure about the pregnancy and didn't anticipate feeling so profoundly about the loss. On the other hand, you may find that others assume you are relieved when, in reality, you are experiencing anything but relief. This discrepancy between your inner emotions and external expectations can be deeply unsettling (*Your Feelings and Emotions After Miscarriage*, 2019).

Loneliness: Navigating Isolation and Relationship Dynamics

Some women find themselves feeling isolated in their grief because nobody knew about their pregnancy in the first place. This isolation can be further compounded if friends, family, or acquaintances react insensitively or dismissively to your loss (*Your Feelings and Emotions After Miscarriage*, 2019). Couples may also experience anxiety about how the miscarriage has affected their relationship with one another. The process of grieving and coping can vary significantly between partners.

Consider whether you might want to confide in your employer, close colleagues, friends, or family members. Sharing your experience can help you feel less isolated and better supported.

One individual reflects on her experience with sharing her loss (*Your Feelings and Emotions After Miscarriage*, 2019):

"I, for one, found the thought of waiting 3 months to tell our families and close friends impossible. The way they shared in our excitement and later our grief really meant something to us. I found it almost impossible to tell anyone at work, so I didn't feel I could share my loss. I had a silent scream in my head I couldn't let out."

Coping Strategies for Healing

While there is no one-size-fits-all approach to coping with the emotions following a miscarriage, there are several practical strategies that can facilitate the healing process (*Your Feelings and Emotions After Miscarriage*, 2019):

- **Allow Yourself to Feel Sad:** Grant yourself permission to grieve. Do not pressure yourself to feel happy, even if a significant amount of time has passed since your miscarriage. Feeling sadness is a healthy part of the grieving process.
- **Commemorate Your Loss:** Many individuals find solace in finding a special way to remember their baby or to create a meaningful ritual to say goodbye. This process can provide a sense of closure and a tangible connection to the lost pregnancy.
- **Express Yourself:** Consider keeping a journal or confiding in a trusted friend, family member, or professional counselor about your emotions. Sharing your feelings can be profoundly therapeutic and assist in processing your grief.
- **Prioritize Self-Care:** Attend to both your physical and emotional health. This includes maintaining a healthy, balanced diet and seeking medical attention if you are struggling with sleep. Emotional stress can lead to exhaustion, so self-care is paramount.
- **Avoid "Numbing" the Pain:** It may be tempting to turn to substances like alcohol or other forms of escape to numb the pain temporarily. However, this approach often intensifies emotional turmoil

when the numbness wears off. It is advisable to refrain from using substances as a coping mechanism.

If Coping Becomes Overwhelming

Sometimes, grief can become all-encompassing, and seeking professional help becomes imperative. Mental health problems may develop as a result of the grief associated with losing a baby (*Your Feelings and Emotions After Miscarriage*, 2019). Depression and anxiety are common reactions, but some individuals may experience more severe conditions, such as post-traumatic stress disorder (PTSD) or perinatal obsessive-compulsive disorder (OCD).

Toni shares her experience: "I struggled with anxiety and felt very low. In fact, I felt like I was losing my mind" (*Your Feelings and Emotions After Miscarriage*, 2019).

If you or someone you know is struggling to cope with the emotional aftermath of a miscarriage, do not hesitate to reach out to a healthcare professional for guidance and support. Mental health issues related to grief are treatable, and there is help available (*Your Feelings and Emotions After Miscarriage*, 2019).

You can also find support through organizations such as Tommy's, which offers free counseling and resources. Their midwives are trained in bereavement support and can provide assistance during difficult times.

Coping with the emotions following a miscarriage is a deeply personal journey, one that requires time, patience, and self-compassion. There is no predetermined timeline for healing, and everyone's experience is unique. It is essential to acknowledge your feelings, seek support when needed, and prioritize self-care during this challenging period.

Remember, you are not alone in your emotions, and there is help available to guide you through this difficult time. Reach out to healthcare professionals, support groups, or organizations specializing in miscarriage and pregnancy loss for the assistance and guidance you require. Healing is possible, and with time, you can find a path toward emotional recovery and acceptance (*Your Feelings and Emotions After Miscarriage*, 2019).

When you are ready to try again—take all the time you need—I want you to focus on the positive steps you can take to provide the best possible environment for your baby—inside your body. In the next chapter, we explore the ways in which we can prepare the body for its delightful guest and ensure that we are in peak health.

8

BLOSSOM

The above chapter title is an acronym: Building Lifestyle Optimization Through Stress Reduction, Sleep, and Mindfulness. It cannot be over-emphasized just how crucial it is that both partners maintain a healthy, fit lifestyle to improve your chances of success. Look at this heart-warming success story following a complete lifestyle change to see what I mean.

ALEIYA AND MICHAL'S STORY

"The journey through infertility is like navigating a labyrinth in the darkest corners of your mind. It's a place where hope often flickers like a fragile flame, and despair lurks around every turn. Our story, Aleiya's and mine was one of such uncertainty until we discovered the guiding light named Julia.

I can't even begin to describe how Julia has helped us. It was a time when we felt lost, adrift in a sea of unanswered questions. A miscarriage had left us shattered, our dreams of parenthood hanging by a thread. We needed answers, but the path forward was shrouded in obscurity. That's when Julia's name found its way into our lives like a whispered secret.

It's funny how life's most significant turning points often come from recommendations, a nod from fate herself. I reached out to Julia, apprehension mingling with hope. Little did we know it would be the best and smartest move we'd make on our fertility journey.

Julia, a beacon of knowledge and compassion, didn't just guide us; she held our hands through the storm. She helped us prepare our bodies, ensuring we were in the best possible shape to embark on this tumultuous journey. Her expertise extended beyond nutrition; she was a compass guiding us to healthcare professionals who could provide the answers we so desperately sought.

In my case, Julia's wisdom led us to the startling revelation of an underactive thyroid. It was something I had never considered, hidden beneath the surface of my daily life, camouflaged by my lack of awareness. But Julia saw what I couldn't, and thanks to her, I embarked on a path to healing.

For my husband, her guidance was equally transformative. She orchestrated semen analyses that uncovered terms foreign to us before our journey: low morphology and DNA fragmentation. Esoteric words that turned out to be pivotal in our quest for parenthood.

I stand here today, 21 weeks pregnant, with gratitude swelling in my heart. Julia, with her tailored, evidence-based nutritional advice, not only prepared us for this miracle but also transformed our overall well-being. People began to notice improvements in my skin and hair, even before pregnancy came into the picture. It was a testament to the power of what we put into our bodies and how it reverberates through every facet of our health.

But Julia isn't just a nutritional therapist; she's a guardian angel on this winding journey. We initially sought her out for dietary guidance and lifestyle changes, but she offered us something more profound. In the labyrinth of fertility, she'd walked the path countless times before. She knew precisely which turn to take, which door to open, to lead us toward our ultimate goal: our baby.

Today, Aleiya and I are forever grateful to Julia. She is the pivotal force behind our journey, the hand that helped us find our way out of the darkness, and the light that guides us toward our dream of becoming parents. Without her, this beautiful chapter in our lives might have remained a distant dream" (Young, n.d.).

THE IMPORTANCE OF A HEALTHY LIFESTYLE

Let me tell you an interesting story. Once upon a time, in a world where smartphones buzzed more often than bees and stress levels soared higher than an eagle with a caffeine addiction, there lived two cheeky characters—Mathias Abiodun Emokpae and Somieye Imaobong Brown. They weren't your ordinary protagonists; they were fertility crusaders on a mission to make the world a more baby-friendly place, one laugh at a time!

Lifestyle Shenanigans and Fertility—The Unlikely Duo

Our story begins with a conundrum. You see, there's this thing called fertility, and it's kind of a big deal for us humans. Without it, the world wouldn't be blessed with adorable baby toes and chubby cheeks. But wait, here's the kicker—our lifestyle choices are doing the cha-cha with our fertility!

Picture this: you're on the dance floor of life, grooving to the rhythm of modifiable lifestyle factors. There's the tempting fat-rich diet, the smooth moves of delayed childbearing, the smoky allure of tobacco, and the wild partners in crime—alcohol misuse and anxiety. These party animals can lead to a fertility fiasco, and trust us, it's not a dance-off you want to win!

The Chain Reaction of Chaos

Now, let's delve deeper into this wild lifestyle party. You've got delayed childbearing, who's like that friend who can't decide between ordering pizza or Chinese for dinner. They're juggling careers and education, and before you know it, they're knocking on the door of forty, wondering where all the good eggs went!

And then there's the infamous couple—Mr. Smoke and Miss Booze. They love to hang out together, sharing laughs and lung damage. But here's the twist: they invite their mischievous friend Anxiety to the party. Together, they create stress, which is like the uninvited guest who spills red wine on your brand-new white carpet.

All this stress and chaos lead to some unhealthy choices. You might find yourself reaching for that extra shot of espresso or sneaking in a few cigarettes, thinking they're your allies. But, oh boy, they're not! They're like the sugar rush before the sugar crash, and the crash isn't pretty.

Saving the Day With Lifestyle Makeovers

But fret not, dear readers, for every wild party has its designated driver. In this case, it's our heroes, Mathias Abiodun Emokpae and Somieye Imaobong Brown. They've gathered evidence from the scientific treasure trove and brought us some practical recommendations.

So, how do we save the day? Well, start by ditching the fat-rich diet for some leafy greens and lean proteins. Let's also put a stop to the career vs. baby tug-of-war and bring balance back into our lives. And as for our wild friends, Smoke and Booze, it's time to show them the exit sign (Emokpae & Brown, 2021).

The Misconception of ART and the Quest for Baby Wisdom

Now, let's talk about the misconceptions. Some folks think ART is like baking a baby in a lab, complete with goggles and a lab coat. But it's not! It's just nature getting a little help from science.

The real key is awareness. We need to spread the word about the causes of infertility and the wonders of in vitro fertilization (Emokpae & Brown, 2021). It's like telling everyone that your favorite dessert place is open around the clock—everyone should know!

It's Time to BLOSSOM

In the end, folks, it's all about making those lifestyle choices that make your body a fertility-friendly wonderland. Say goodbye to stress, bad diets, and poor fitness. Say hello to a world where babies bloom like beautiful flowers.

So, let's all join hands (not too tightly, though; we don't want to crush any fertility vibes) and pledge to live life with a little more laughter, a little less stress, and a whole lot of love. It's time to BLOSSOM and make this world a better place for future generations!

And that, my friends, is the story of how lifestyle choices and fertility became unlikely dance partners in the grand ball of life. So, go forth, make those healthy choices, and let's keep the baby-making dance floor bustling with joy and laughter!

OBESITY AND EATING DISORDERS: A WEIGHTY MATTER FOR FERTILITY

In today's world, we're presented with an abundance of culinary temptations, often high in calories but lacking essential nutrients. This phenomenon has contributed to a global rise in obesity, and interestingly, it's not just our waistlines that are affected.

Obesity isn't merely a concern for our physical health; it's a significant factor impacting reproductive health as well. High-fat diets can tinker with the physical and molecular structure of sperm cells, disrupting their vitality and DNA integrity. Studies involving mice showed that indulging in high-fat diets led to long-term alterations in the reproductive system. This included changes in the seminiferous epithelium and seminiferous tubules, ultimately resulting in decreased sperm concentration and quality (Emokpae & Brown, 2021).

Furthermore, obesity has a substantial impact on hormonal balance. Excess body fat can disrupt the delicate hormonal equilibrium of the reproductive system. This hormonal chaos can lead to conditions like PCOS and metabolic syndrome, which in turn can hinder fertility (Emokpae & Brown, 2021).

So, it's not just about shedding pounds for aesthetic reasons; maintaining a healthy weight is crucial for fertility. A diet rich in fruits, vegetables, legumes, and fish has been linked to better sperm quality and lower DNA fragmentation (Emokpae & Brown, 2021). Conversely, frequent consumption of red meat has been associated with lower sperm quality.

Eating Disorders: A Battle of Body and Mind

On the flip side, eating disorders such as Bulimia nervosa and Anorexia nervosa can cast a shadow over fertility dreams, especially in women. Bulimia nervosa is characterized by binge eating followed by behaviors like fasting or purging, driven by an obsessive desire to lose weight. Anorexia nervosa, on the other hand, involves extreme self-starvation due to a distorted body image (Emokpae & Brown, 2021).

These disorders can suppress ovulation, leaving women struggling with infertility. In fact, they account for up to 60% of cases of anovulatory infertility (Emokpae & Brown, 2021). The good news is that the likelihood of a cure is higher with Bulimia nervosa, emphasizing the importance of early intervention and support.

NUTRITIONAL ALTITUDE AND SPERM QUALITY

Men, too, need to be mindful of their dietary choices. Emerging evidence suggests a direct link between nutrition and semen quality (Emokpae & Brown, 2021). High-fat diets can wreak havoc on not only sperm cells but also fetal development.

Intriguingly, studies involving rodents showed that high-fat diets resulted in testicular alterations, decreased sperm concentration, and DNA integrity. Normal testicular function is highly responsive to changes in overall metabolism. Thus, a high-energy diet can influence testicular metabolism, potentially affecting fertility (Emokpae & Brown, 2021).

On the bright side, research suggests that making dietary modifications, including increasing the consumption of fruits, vegetables, legumes, and fish, can enhance reproductive health (Emokpae & Brown, 2021). These foods have been associated with better sperm quality and a lower DNA fragmentation index.

The Three Culprits: Smoking, Alcohol, and Caffeine

Now, let's discuss three notorious culprits: smoking, alcohol, and caffeine. These substances have a profound impact on fertility and deserve our close attention.

Smoking: A Fertility Killer

Cigarette smoking is not only harmful to your lungs but also to your reproductive health. It can reduce sperm concentration, damage sperm DNA, and impair sperm motility in men. In women, smoking can lead to a thicker zona pellucida, making it harder for sperm to penetrate eggs (Emokpae & Brown, 2021). Furthermore, menopause tends to occur earlier in smoking women.

The detrimental effects of smoking on fertility are primarily attributed to the toxic substances in tobacco smoke, including nicotine, cadmium, lead, and free radicals (Emokpae & Brown, 2021). These culprits can cause oxidative stress and DNA damage.

The good news is that quitting smoking can significantly improve fertility outcomes. Every year of smoking cessation can reduce the risk of ART failure by four percent, especially during the critical stages of clinical pregnancy to live birth (Emokpae & Brown, 2021).

Alcohol: A Double-Edged Sword

While alcohol is often associated with celebration and relaxation, excessive consumption can be detrimental to fertility. Alcohol depletes essential nutrients from the body, disrupts hormonal balance, and may lead to amenorrhea in women. In men, chronic alcohol consumption can lower testosterone levels, impair sperm count and motility, and alter testicular morphology (Emokpae & Brown, 2021).

Notably, high alcohol consumption during pregnancy can increase the risk of low birth weight, birth defects, and miscarriage (Emokpae & Brown, 2021). It's advisable for individuals trying to conceive to either abstain from alcohol or limit their consumption significantly.

Caffeine: The Silent Disruptor

Caffeine, a ubiquitous stimulant found in coffee, tea, soft drinks, and chocolate, can have a significant impact on fertility. High caffeine intake exceeding 500 mg per day has been associated with delayed pregnancy by interrupting the fertilization and implantation process (Emokpae & Brown, 2021).

Pregnant women, in particular, are advised to avoid caffeine altogether due to its potential to harm the fetus. Although there's no definitive safe level of caffeine consumption, moderation is key for those trying to conceive, pregnant, or breastfeeding (Emokpae & Brown, 2021).

PHYSICAL EXERCISE: BALANCING ACT

Exercise undoubtedly benefits overall health, but it's essential to strike the right balance. Rigorous physical activity can lead to energy imbalances, potentially causing amenorrhea and irregular ovulation in women (Emokpae

& Brown, 2021). For overweight or obese women, exercise combined with weight loss can improve fertility.

In contrast, a sedentary lifestyle can also have adverse effects on fertility, as biological evidence supports the association between physical activity and infertility. The key lies in moderation and a balanced approach to exercise (Emokpae & Brown, 2021).

Sexual Behavior: A Matter of Health and Safety

Promiscuity, while a personal choice, can increase the risk of sexually transmitted infections (STIs). These infections can lead to infertility, both in men and women. Early diagnosis and treatment of STIs are essential to prevent their adverse effects on reproductive health (Emokpae & Brown, 2021).

Drug Abuse: A Threat to Fertility

Drug abuse is a significant concern, affecting both women and men differently. Heroin and methadone can cause amenorrhea in women, while substances like marijuana, heroin, methamphetamine, and cocaine can disrupt hormonal balance and impair reproductive function in both genders (Emokpae & Brown, 2021). Avoiding illicit drug use is crucial for preserving fertility.

Cellular Phones and Radiation: A Silent Threat

The ever-increasing use of cellular phones has raised concerns about their potential impact on fertility. Mobile phones emit radiation that can harm sperm motility, number, and morphology. While more research is needed, it's advisable to exercise caution and limit prolonged exposure to cell phone radiation, especially when storing phones in trouser pockets (Emokpae & Brown, 2021).

In the grand tapestry of life, the threads of nutrition and lifestyle choices intricately weave the patterns of fertility. By making informed decisions and embracing a balanced approach to nutrition and lifestyle, we can nurture the fertile soil in which the seeds of parenthood can flourish. Remember, life's journey to parenthood is a remarkable one, and every choice we make can shape the destination. So, let's tread with care, nurturing the dream of parenthood every step of the way.

THE INVISIBLE CULPRITS: ANXIETY, DEPRESSION, AND MISCONCEPTION

While we've been navigating the labyrinth of lifestyle choices and nutritional factors impacting fertility, there are some intangible yet equally potent forces at play. Anxiety, depression, and misconceptions can cast a shadow over the path to parenthood (Emokpae & Brown, 2021).

The Silent Suffering: Anxiety and Depression

In the colorful tapestry of human emotions, anxiety and depression are shades that can dim the vibrant desire for parenthood. In Nigeria, where procreation often carries societal significance, the inability to achieve this cherished goal can lead to marital discord and emotional turmoil (Emokpae & Brown, 2021).

Studies have shown that almost half of infertile women in Nigeria experience psychiatric morbidity. The absence of support, unfair treatment, discrimination, and induced abortion are often more prevalent among infertile women (Emokpae & Brown, 2021). Anxiety and depression can take root in this soil of despair, affecting not just mental health but also reproductive health.

For men, anxiety and depression can also have a profound impact, particularly on spermatogenesis—the complex interplay of hormones in the hypothalamic-pituitary-adrenal (HPA) axis can disrupt testosterone secretion, affecting sperm production. This hormonal cascade can lead to changes in Sertoli cells, and the blood test is a barrier, ultimately halting the journey of sperm (Emokpae & Brown, 2021).

For women, the story is similar, with the hypothalamic-pituitary-gonadal (HPG) axis bearing the brunt of anxiety and depression. Corticotropin-releasing hormone (CRH) can inhibit hypothalamic GnRH secretion, while glucocorticoids can disrupt hormonal balance, potentially leading to 'hypothalamic' amenorrhea (Emokpae & Brown, 2021).

The lesson here is clear: stress management is crucial for couples striving to conceive. Periodic relaxation activities can be a soothing balm on the path to parenthood.

Misconceptions and Beliefs: The Invisible Hurdles

In the rich tapestry of human culture, misconceptions and beliefs are threads that can either weave a tapestry of hope or cast a shadow of doubt. In many developing countries, particularly in West Africa, myths about infertility abound.

Some believe infertility is the result of evil spirits, a predestined fate, or a punishment from a higher power (Emokpae & Brown, 2021). These misconceptions can be deeply ingrained, often requiring prayers and patience to resolve, or so they believe.

But science paints a different picture. Advances in medical sciences have shown that infertility is not a curse or a supernatural challenge; it's a medical condition with treatment options. Assisted reproductive technologies, such as IVF, offer hope to those struggling with infertility. However, misconceptions persist, labeling IVF as unnatural and culturally inappropriate (Emokpae & Brown, 2021).

This misunderstanding has led to a clandestine approach to ART treatment in Nigeria, driven by the fear of stigmatization. Lack of awareness and these beliefs further hinder access to infertility treatment, especially among the uneducated.

Even among the educated, strong family support systems can delay the decision to seek treatment, with many opting to "wait on God" for a natural conception.

A Call to Action: Education and Awareness

To untangle this web of misconceptions and beliefs, education and awareness are key. Reproductive health education can shed light on the true causes of infertility and the importance of IVF and other treatments. Public health campaigns should intensify efforts to educate about the harmful effects of substance abuse and misconceptions (Emokpae & Brown, 2021).

Legislation and enforcement of laws regulating drug and substance abuse can also play a role in mitigating these negative influences on individuals and society. In the intricate dance of fertility, anxiety, depression, and misconceptions may lurk in the shadows. But armed with knowledge, awareness, and the determination to embrace a healthy lifestyle, couples can brighten the path to parenthood and, in doing so, create the future they desire (Emokpae & Brown, 2021).

So, let's navigate this final leg of the journey with clarity, hope, and the conviction that parenthood is a dream worth pursuing, no matter what challenges may arise along the way.

Course of Action: Get Your Health on Track for Fertility

Deciding to embark on the journey of parenthood is a thrilling chapter in anyone's life. However, when the stork takes a little longer than expected to knock on your door, it can be a tad frustrating. Fear not, though, for science and lifestyle changes are here to lend a hand. So, if you're ready to take those steps toward parenthood, let's dive into an eight-step course of action for boosting your fertility (Paciuc, n.d.).

Step 1: Understand Infertility

First things first, let's get familiar with the concept. Infertility is when you've been engaging in the baby-making dance for a year without any positive results (or six months if you're over 35). There can be many culprits behind infertility, from hormonal imbalances to structural quirks in your reproductive system. Dr. John Paciuc, our seasoned infertility specialist in New York City, can be your guide in deciphering the puzzle of infertility.

Step 2: Use Sperm-Friendly Lubricant

Let's start with a simple yet vital change—your choice of lubricant. Some lubes have spermicides that could throw a wrench in your conception plans. Opt for a lube that's gentle on those little swimmers to keep the path to fertilization clear and obstacle-free.

Step 3: Track Your Cycle

Getting cozy with your menstrual cycle can be a game-changer. By tracking it, you can pinpoint those golden days when conception is most likely. Keep an eye out for fertile cervical mucus or even use ovulation confirmation strips—they work just like pregnancy tests and are easy peasy to use).

Step 4: Maintain a Healthy Weight

Want a tip that's as straightforward as it gets? Keep your weight in check. Being on the heavier side can mess with your hormone balance, leading to irregular ovulation. So, shed those extra pounds and give your body a better shot at fertility.

Step 5: Kick the Smoking Habit

Cigarette smoke isn't just the enemy of your lungs; it's no friend to your eggs either. Smoking can harm egg quality, so if you're planning to become a parent, consider quitting this habit pronto.

Step 6: Moderate Alcohol Intake

Cheers to moderation! Consuming more than four servings of alcohol a day can do a number on both male and female fertility. So, if you're fond of the occasional tipple, it might be time to cut back while you're on the road to conception.

Step 7: Keep Caffeine in Check

For all you coffee enthusiasts out there, I've got a nugget I think you should know: too much caffeine, more than 200 mg a day, could up your chances of an early miscarriage. So, while you're preparing for parenthood, consider tweaking your caffeine intake.

Step 8: Zen Out and Prioritize Sleep

Last but not least, don't underestimate the power of stress management and a good night's sleep. Excess stress can throw a wrench into your fertility plans, and poor sleep can do the same. Incorporate deep breathing, meditation, or perhaps a calming yoga session into your routine. Also, aim for seven to nine hours of quality sleep each night.

There you have it—an eight-step roadmap to whip your health into tip-top fertility shape. Remember, you're not alone on this journey. As you embark on this path to parenthood, do it with a smile and a sense of hope because your journey is just beginning, and brighter days are on the horizon!

DESTRESSING WHEN YOU'RE TRYING TO CONCEIVE

The pursuit of parenthood is a profound journey laden with emotions, and sometimes, the road can feel endlessly winding. The anticipation, the two-week waiting period, and the cyclical nature of trying can become emotionally taxing. While well-intentioned advice suggests that "just relaxing will do the trick," we understand it's not that simple. In this section, we will delve into expert-backed methods to help you effectively manage stress during your quest to conceive.

The Power of Journaling

Keeping a brutally honest journal can be a therapeutic release for your emotions. This practice goes beyond documenting your day; it's about giving voice to complex and sometimes negative thoughts that might be weighing on your mind. Research shows that journaling can prevent rumination—a process of repeatedly mulling over negative thoughts, which can lead to depression and anxiety (Mauer, 2020).

Connect with Supportive Friends

After you've poured your thoughts into your journal, reach out to a trusted friend. Choose someone who excels in lending a compassionate ear but won't encourage you to dwell on worries. Sharing your feelings with a confidant can be remarkably soothing (Mauer, 2020).

Harness the Power of TTC Tools

Understanding the intricacies of your menstrual cycle and fertility is crucial for optimizing your chances of conceiving. Tracking ovulation through kits or basal body temperature thermometers is a proactive approach that empowers you with knowledge, alleviating stress caused by uncertainty (Mauer, 2020).

Embrace the Great Outdoors

Spending time in natural surroundings is linked to reduced rates of depression and anxiety. Plan outdoor activities with your partner, not only for the benefits of fresh air but also to strengthen your bond. Focusing on shared experiences rather than fertility struggles can offer respite (Mauer, 2020).

Find Solace in a Personal Mantra

For those with spiritual inclinations, creating a personal mantra can be a powerful stress-relief tool. Studies have demonstrated that repeating a spiritually meaningful phrase can effectively alleviate anxiety and insomnia (Mauer, 2020). Choose a mantra that resonates with you, promoting calm and tranquility.

Soothe Your Soul With a Swim

Consider indulging in saltwater therapy if the opportunity arises. Studies reveal that floating in saltwater triggers the body's relaxation response, reducing stress hormone levels (Mauer, 2020). Regular relaxation in floating tanks has been associated with better sleep, improved optimism, and decreased anxiety, stress, and depression.

Harness Positive Language

Maintain an optimistic approach in your discussions and self-reflection. Adopting an "optimistic explanatory style" has been proven to enhance one's outlook (Mauer, 2020). Rather than framing thoughts negatively, focus on your proactive efforts and reassure yourself that you are doing everything in your power.

Exercise Mindfully

Regular physical activity is a well-acknowledged stress reliever. Engage in exercise routines you enjoy but remember not to overexert yourself. Excessive vigorous exercise can potentially disrupt ovulation (Mauer, 2020). Listen to your body, as it will guide you on the right balance.

The Power of Taking a Break

If the relentless pursuit of conception is becoming all-encompassing, it's perfectly acceptable to take a step back. Communicate with your partner and decide to take a break from trying to conceive. Redirect your energy toward other passions and interests, such as signing up for a race, planning a road trip, or engaging in volunteer work (Mauer, 2020). Sometimes, clearing your mind can yield significant benefits.

Prioritize "Me" Time

Amidst the hustle and bustle of daily life, make it a point to allocate time solely for yourself. Research from the University of Sussex highlights the stress-reducing benefits of activities such as reading, listening to music, or enjoying a cup of tea (Mauer, 2020). Just six minutes of reading can lower heart rate and reduce tension.

Rediscover the Joy of Intimacy

Remember the person beside you, the one you're embarking on this journey with. Set aside moments for meaningful couple time that doesn't revolve around tracking cervical mucus or ovulation calendars (Mauer, 2020). Plan dates, enjoy activities, and even watch a comedy show together. Anticipating laughter has the power to decrease stress hormone levels.

While the road to conception may be fraught with challenges, it's essential to prioritize your emotional well-being. These strategies offer a comprehensive toolkit to effectively manage stress as you navigate the path to parenthood. Remember, you are not alone in this journey, and by incorporating these techniques, you can find balance, tranquility, and joy amidst the pursuit of your ultimate goal: becoming a parent.

When the stars align, the universe hears your fervent prayers and affirmation, and the magic descends into your receptive womb, you will know that all that effort, hard work, and determination was worth it. And that is where the real work begins. It will take the greatest care and attention to get you through that tricky first trimester.

THE BEGINNING—THE FIRST TRIMESTER EXPERIENCE

I wish I could tell you that once you conceive, all your troubles will disappear, and it will be nothing but rainbows and sunshine from here on out. And, for some couples, it does pan out that way. However, for a staggering number of couples, pregnancy proves to be much more of a challenge than conception. Take a look at the following story to see just what I mean.

EMMA'S MIRACLE: OUR JOURNEY OF HOPE

"Becoming a mother to our daughter, Emma, was a dream that Eric and I held close to our hearts. It's a dream we now fondly call our "miracle" because the path we traveled to parenthood was filled with challenges, determination, and the exceptional care we received from Sutter Health.

Our journey began with three emotionally taxing years of in vitro fertilization and three heartbreaking miscarriages. Each loss was a painful reminder of our deep desire to become parents, a dream that sometimes felt like it was slipping away.

Amidst our struggles, we found a glimmer of hope at Sutter Health, where compassionate caregivers would become our guiding lights. Little did we know that the most challenging part of our journey was yet to come.

Around the three-month mark of what seemed like a typical pregnancy, my world was rocked by alarming bleeding. Dr. Deborah Shapiro, a name forever etched in our hearts, admitted me to Peninsula Medical Center for exploratory surgery. What unfolded during that surgery was both heartbreaking and life-saving.

I had been carrying twins, a revelation that filled us with joy and anticipation. However, one of our precious babies had implanted in my fallopian tube, leading to a rupture—an ectopic pregnancy that threatened both our lives. Dr. Shapiro made the agonizing decision to remove the ectopic embryo, a moment that mixed sorrow with gratitude as one life was lost, and another continued to flourish.

Our journey was not without further challenges. Weeks later, our hearts were gripped by fear as we struggled to detect our baby's heartbeat. An immediate ultrasound became our lifeline, and it was during that anxious moment that our miracle happened.

The ultrasound technician's voice filled the room with excitement, and tears of joy replaced those of despair. On the screen, we witnessed our little Emma waving her tiny hand, a poignant message of hope and life. From that moment on, I spent the rest of my pregnancy on bed rest, nurturing our precious miracle.

Two weeks before Emma's official due date, she arrived, perfectly healthy, and our family was complete. Throughout our journey, we were surrounded by dedicated professionals who made us feel like we were the only ones that mattered.

Our story is a testament to the power of hope, unwavering support, and the incredible strength of families. Emma's arrival is a cherished moment, a symbol of the love that carried us through our journey of trials and tribulations" (*Miracle Baby Born After Difficult Pregnancy*, n.d.).

EARLY PREGNANCY SYMPTOMS AND CHANGES

Are you ready for the exhilarating journey of pregnancy? Even before that missed period, the signs and symptoms of pregnancy can drop subtle hints of the incredible life-changing event that might be in store for you (Mayo

Clinic Staff, 2021). Let's explore these early signs and why they occur as you embark on this exciting adventure.

Classic Signs and Symptoms

- **Missed Period:** Perhaps this is the most obvious sign. If your expected menstrual cycle is delayed by a week or more, especially if you have a regular cycle, it's time to consider the possibility of pregnancy.
- **Tender, Swollen Breasts:** In the early stages, hormonal changes can make your breasts sensitive and sore. But fear not, this discomfort typically eases off as your body adjusts to the hormonal shifts.
- **Nausea and Vomiting:** Ah, morning sickness! Contrary to its name, it can strike any time of the day or night. For many women, it starts a month or two after conception, but each pregnancy is unique. While the exact cause remains a mystery, pregnancy hormones are believed to play a significant role.
- **Increased Urination:** Are you suddenly finding yourself making more trips to the bathroom than usual? That's because your body's blood volume increases during pregnancy, leading your kidneys to process extra fluids that end up in your bladder.
- **Fatigue:** Are you feeling inexplicably tired? You're not alone. The surge in the hormone progesterone

during early pregnancy can leave you feeling exhausted, even if you've had a good night's sleep.

Other Signs and Symptoms

- **Moodiness:** Blame it on the hormones! The early stages of pregnancy can unleash a flood of emotions, making you more emotional and prone to mood swings.
- **Bloating:** Hormonal shifts can cause bloating, akin to how you feel during your menstrual cycle.
- **Light Spotting:** Sometimes, a hint of blood can be one of the earliest signs of pregnancy. Known as implantation bleeding, it occurs when the fertilized egg attaches to the uterine lining around 10 to 14 days post-conception.
- **Cramping:** Some women experience mild uterine cramping in the early stages.
- **Constipation:** Hormonal changes can slow down your digestive system, potentially leading to constipation.
- **Food Aversions:** Your sense of smell and taste may become more sensitive during pregnancy, leading to changes in food preferences—blame it on those hormones again!
- **Nasal Congestion:** Increasing hormone levels and blood production can cause your nasal membranes to swell and dry out, sometimes resulting in a stuffy or runny nose.

Are You Really Pregnant?

While these signs and symptoms are promising indicators of pregnancy, they aren't exclusive to it. Some could hint at other factors, such as illness or an impending period. Nonetheless, if you miss a period and notice these signs, consider taking a home pregnancy test or consulting your healthcare provider (Mayo Clinic Staff, 2021). Confirming your pregnancy early allows you to kickstart essential prenatal care, ensuring the best start for you and your growing little one.

Whether you're planning to conceive or have just received the exciting news, consider embracing a daily prenatal vitamin (Mayo Clinic Staff, 2021). These supplements, packed with crucial vitamins and minerals like folic acid and iron, support your baby's healthy growth and development.

The pregnancy journey is awe-inspiring, filled with surprises, challenges, and boundless joy. Embrace it, celebrate it, and savor every moment as you step into the incredible world of motherhood.

PREGNANCY MYTHS: DEBUNKING THE BUMPS

Pregnancy, that beautiful journey into motherhood, often comes with its own set of myths and tales. While some may make you raise an eyebrow, others might have you second-guessing your choices (Hetrick, 2022).

Myth #1: Predicting Baby's Gender

From high or low baby bumps to sweet versus salty cravings, many swear by these tricks. But science says, "Hold on!" The only surefire gender reveal is through ultrasound or specific blood tests. Those cravings? Well, maybe your baby just has a diverse palate!

Myth #2: Exercise Exile

Think pregnancy means a workout exile? Think again! Listen to your body and keep your routines going. Just avoid acrobatics unless you're training to become a circus mom!

Myth #3: Let's Talk About Sex, Baby

Concerned about intimacy during pregnancy? Worry not; it's typically safe. In fact, it might even give your cervix a pep talk! Remember, check with your healthcare provider, but keep the sparks flying if you fancy.

Myth #4: Color Conundrum

Want a new hair color to match your pregnancy glow? Go ahead! But maybe wait until after the first trimester—you know, just to be safe. You're the canvas; paint it when you're ready.

Myth #5: The Hot Tub Tango

Hot tubs are a no-go, right? Well, if it's hotter than 101 °F, it's a hard pass. Keep cool, stay hydrated, and don't turn into a human lobster!

Myth #6: The Umbilical Limbo

Ever heard that lifting your arms means the umbilical cord becomes a jump rope? It's true, but here's the kicker: it rarely causes harm. Four out of ten babies are born with a cord twist, and they're just doing the cha-cha in there!

Myth #7: The "Eating for Two" Feast

Newsflash: You're not running a buffet! "Eating for two" is a catchy phrase, but it's a trap. Think quality, not quantity. An extra 300 calories a day is fine, not the entire menu, please!

Myth #8: Coffee Catastrophe

Caffeine addicts, rejoice! You don't have to say goodbye; just limit your intake. Sip wisely; your daily latte isn't going anywhere.

Myth #9: Culinary Caution

Seafood, soft cheese, deli meat, and rare steak—are they off the menu? Not entirely. Just choose wisely; salmon and sushi could still be your pals. Heat soft cheese and deli treats for that extra safety dance.

Myth #10: Heartburn = Baby's Hair?

Prepare for this hairy situation: heartburn doesn't equal a hairy baby. Your heartburn is more like a sneak preview of your baby's fiery personality!

Moms-to-be need to take pregnancy myths with a pinch of humor. Trust your doctor and reliable sources for guidance (Hetrick, 2022). And remember, while these myths might give you a chuckle, your journey to motherhood is unique and magical—just like you!

YOUR FIRST DOCTOR'S APPOINTMENT

The moment you discover you're expecting, a whirlwind of emotions sweeps over you. Excitement, wonder, and perhaps a hint of nervousness dance in your thoughts. Amidst this incredible journey, your first prenatal visit emerges as a beacon of guidance and assurance.

Embarking on the Journey: The Ideal Timing

Your initial prenatal appointment typically falls around the six to eight-week mark (Tabackman, 2021). However, there might be exceptions if you have existing medical conditions, past pregnancy challenges, or unusual symptoms. It's a date marked not just on your calendar but also in your heart—the first step in nurturing the life growing within.

The Essentials: What to Expect

Your first prenatal visit is a comprehensive exploration, both medically and emotionally. It's about more than just your vital signs (Tabackman, 2021). Therefore, you should know what you can anticipate going in.

- **Vital Signs:** Your body's orchestra plays its symphony of life through vital signs like heart rate, breathing rate, and blood pressure. Your last menstrual period helps set the stage, assisting in the calculation of your due date.
- **Reproductive History:** Your doctor seeks insights into your reproductive journey. Past pregnancies, miscarriages, and delivery methods—these details shape your unique path. They guide your doctor in predicting future pregnancy outcomes and personalizing your care.
- **Gynecologic History:** Your gynecological history is a vital piece of the puzzle. Any previous issues, sexually transmitted infections, and Pap smear results become chapters in your story. It's about ensuring a smooth path ahead for both you and your baby.
- **Medical History:** Diseases can cast shadows, but your doctor is here to shine a light. Conditions like diabetes, heart disease, or psychiatric disorders are key players. Knowledge empowers, and close monitoring ensures a safe journey.

- **Family History:** Your family's tale holds invaluable clues. Genetic or inherited conditions peek from the branches of your family tree. Ethnic heritage matters, too, as it can affect your risk profile for certain conditions like diabetes or high blood pressure.

The Golden Thread: Genetic Counseling

For those at risk of specific genetic diseases, genetic counseling offers clarity. This involves an in-depth exploration of your medical history, your partner's, and your family's. Blood tests may be recommended, providing insights into your genetic landscape (Tabackman, 2021).

The Hands-On Approach: Physical Examination

Your first prenatal visit includes a thorough physical exam. It's about more than just the numbers; it's about your well-being. A pelvic exam ensures the health of your pelvis and uterus, while blood and urine tests can uncover crucial information (Tabackman, 2021).

Embrace the Magic: Ultrasound

Depending on your pregnancy's stage, an ultrasound might be your first peek at your little one. It's not just about confirming gestational age; it's that magical moment when a fluttering heart reinforces your love's existence (Tabackman, 2021).

A Careful Peek: Pelvic Exam and Pap Smear

These steps ensure everything's in order within your pelvic region. A Pap smear, though slightly uncomfortable, is a guardian against cervical changes that could lead to cancer (Tabackman, 2021).

The Closing Act: Planning for Tomorrow

As your first prenatal visit concludes, your doctor illuminates the path forward. Additional tests, prenatal vitamins, and valuable advice for a comfortable pregnancy journey take center stage (Tabackman, 2021).

The Frequency of Care: Nurturing Life Month by Month

Throughout your pregnancy, prenatal visits become a cherished rhythm. The first trimester brings monthly checkups, increasing in frequency as you progress. If circumstances require, your doctor will provide extra support.

Your first prenatal visit is not just a medical appointment; it's an embrace of new beginnings. It's about nurturing the promise of life, safeguarding your well-being, and celebrating the unique journey ahead. Embrace it with open arms and cherish every step, for it's a testament to the love that already surrounds your growing family.

Keeping the Game Alive

Now you have everything you need to embark on your fertility journey, it's time to pass on your newfound knowledge and help others find their way.

Simply by sharing your honest thoughts about this book on Amazon, you'll guide other hopeful individuals on their own fertility adventures and kindle their passion for reproductive health.

Thank you for your support. The realm of fertility is enriched when we share our experiences – and your input is an invaluable part of that mission.

Scan the QR code to leave your review on Amazon.

Your participation ensures that the journey for others is illuminated. You're making a difference by sharing your thoughts.

Warm regards,
Kasia Marshall

CONCLUSION

In the tapestry of life, threads of tears and heartache are woven alongside strands of joy and exuberance. The fertility journey, unique to each couple, is a testament to the human spirit's ability to withstand the most profound challenges and emerge stronger than ever before.

We've witnessed countless success stories, each one a beacon of hope in a world of uncertainty. The highs, oh, those glorious highs, where the universe seemed to conspire in our favor. We danced with elation, knowing that our dreams were within reach. Those moments of triumph reminded us that anything was possible. Yet, we also encountered the depths of grief, the lows that threatened to consume us. The tears shed in those moments were not in vain; they were the price we paid for our unwavering determination. We faced setbacks and disappointments, but we never let them define us.

The courage it took to get back up, to want to try again, that courage was our greatest weapon. It was our reminder that, despite the odds, we were not willing to surrender our dreams. We carried our hearts, bruised but resilient, into the battlefield of fertility, ready to fight for the family we envisioned. Through it all, we developed an unshakable resilience, a determination that refused to be silenced. We understood that success demanded more than wishful thinking; it required practical effort, unwavering faith, and a willingness to adapt.

We learned that the journey to parenthood was not a straight path but a winding road with unexpected twists and turns. It was a journey that tested our patience, strained our relationships, and challenged our beliefs. Yet, amid uncertainty, we found strength within ourselves and within each other. The importance of never giving up cannot be overstated. We saw couples who faced seemingly insurmountable odds, who weathered storm after storm, and who, against all odds, emerged as parents. Their stories were a testament to the indomitable human spirit.

In this journey, we discovered that while we couldn't control every outcome, we could control our determination. We could choose hope, even in the face of despair. We could find solace in the arms of our partners, our pillars of support. And now, as we stand at the end of this path, looking back at the trials and tribulations we've overcome, we realize that we've won in the most profound way. Our resilience, our determination, and our love have brought us here.

For those who continue to walk this journey, know that your story is still being written. The tears and heartache, the joy and exuberance, are all part of your unique narrative. Embrace the highs, endure the lows, and never underestimate the strength that resides within you.

In the end, it's not just about conceiving a child; it's about birthing a family and nurturing a love that can withstand any challenge. Your journey is a testament to the beauty of the human spirit, the power of unwavering hope, and the resilience of the heart.

So, dear fellow travelers on this winding road, keep moving forward with courage in your hearts and love as your guide. Your destination may still be on the horizon, but with each step, you are one step closer to holding your precious miracle in your arms.

And if this book has given you any comfort, hope, courage, or knowledge on your journey, its purpose having then been served, I thank you for your kindness in leaving a favorable review.

GLOSSARY

Basal Body Temperature (BBT)	The temperature of the body at rest.
Birth Control	Devices or medications used to prevent pregnancy.
Endometriosis	A condition in which tissue that lines the uterus is found outside of the uterus, usually on the ovaries, fallopian tubes, and other pelvic structures.
Fallopian Tubes	Tubes through which an egg travels from the ovary to the uterus.
Follicles	The sac-like structures in which eggs develop inside the ovary.
Hormones	Substances made in the body that control the function of cells or organs.
Hysterosalpingography	A special X-ray procedure in which a small amount of fluid is placed into the uterus and fallopian tubes to find abnormal changes or to see if the tubes are blocked.
Hysteroscopy	A procedure in which a lighted telescope is inserted into the uterus through the cervix to view the inside of the uterus or perform surgery.
Infertility	The inability to get pregnant after 1 year of having regular sexual intercourse without the use of birth control.
Laparoscopy	A surgical procedure in which a thin, lighted telescope called a laparoscope is inserted through a small incision (cut) in the abdomen. The laparoscope is used to view the pelvic organs. Other instruments can be used with it to perform surgery.

Luteinizing Hormone (LH)	A hormone made in the pituitary gland that helps an egg to be released from the ovary.
Menstrual Cycle	The monthly process of changes that occur to prepare a woman's body for possible pregnancy. A menstrual cycle is defined as the first day of menstrual bleeding of one cycle to the first day of menstrual bleeding of the next cycle.
Obstetrician–Gynecologist (Ob-Gyn)	A doctor with special training and education in women's health.
Ovaries	Organs in women that contain the eggs necessary to get pregnant and make important hormones, such as estrogen, progesterone, and testosterone.
Ovulation	The time when an ovary releases an egg.
Pituitary Gland	A gland located near the brain that controls growth and other changes in the body.
Progesterone	A female hormone that is made in the ovaries and prepares the lining of the uterus for pregnancy.
Reproductive Endocrinologist	An obstetrician–gynecologist with special training to manage disorders related to hormones of the reproductive system. These specialists also treat infertility.
Scrotum	The external genital sac in the male that contains the testicles.
Semen	The fluid made by male sex glands that contain sperm.
Sexual Intercourse	The act of the penis of the male entering the vagina of the female. Also called "having sex" or "making love").

Sexually Transmitted Infections (STIs)	Infections that are spread by sexual contact. Infections include chlamydia, gonorrhea, human papillomavirus (HPV), herpes, syphilis, and human immunodeficiency virus (HIV, the cause of acquired immunodeficiency syndrome [AIDS]).
Sonohysterography	A procedure in which sterile fluid is injected into the uterus through the cervix while ultrasound images are taken of the inside of the uterus.
Sperm	A cell produced in the male testicles that can fertilize a female egg.
Testicles	Paired male organs that produce sperm and the male sex hormone testosterone. Also called "testes."
Thyroid Gland	A butterfly-shaped gland located at the base of the neck in front of the windpipe. This gland makes, stores, and releases thyroid hormone, which controls the body's metabolism and regulates how parts of the body work.
Ultrasound Exam	A test in which sound waves are used to examine inner parts of the body. During pregnancy, ultrasound can be used to check the fetus.
Urologist	A physician who specializes in treating problems of the kidneys, bladder, and male reproductive system.
Uterus	A muscular organ in the female pelvis. During pregnancy, this organ holds and nourishes the fetus.

REFERENCES

The benefits of exercising/being active when trying to conceive. (n.d.). Tommy's. https://www.tommys.org/pregnancy-information/planning-a-pregnancy/are-you-ready-to-conceive/being-active-when-trying-conceive

CDC. (2018, January 23). *Planning for pregnancy.* Centers for Disease Control and Prevention. https://www.cdc.gov/preconception/planning.html

Centers for Disease Control and Prevention. (2019). *Infertility.* Centers for Disease Control and Prevention. https://www.cdc.gov/reproductivehealth/infertility/index.htm

Clearblue. (2021, July 8). *Clearblue kinder - Molly's story.* YouTube. https://www.youtube.com/watch?v=uMrpzommDO4&ab_channel=Clearblue

Emokpae, M. A., & Brown, S. I. (2021). Effects of lifestyle factors on fertility: Practical recommendations for modification. *Reproduction and Fertility, 2*(1), R13–R26. https://doi.org/10.1530/RAF-20-0046

Emotional and psychological aspects of fertility treatment. (2023, June 19). GENESIS Fertility Health. https://www.genesisfertility.com/blog/emotional-and-psychological-aspects-of-fertility-treatment/

Evaluating infertility. (2020, January). ACOG. https://www.acog.org/womens-health/faqs/evaluating-infertility

Female infertility. (2022). Penn Medicine. https://www.pennmedicine.org/for-patients-and-visitors/patient-information/conditions-treated-a-to-z/female-infertility

Fertility is a journey, and after two and a half years, here's mine. (2021, May 5). Live Healthy . https://livehealthy.muhealth.org/stories/fertility-journey-and-after-two-and-half-years-heres-mine

Folate and pregnancy. (2019). Pregnancy Birth & Baby. https://www.pregnancybirthbaby.org.au/folate-and-pregnancy

Guttusso, A. N. (2011, July 19). *Success stories after having trouble getting pregnant*. Parents. https://www.parents.com/getting-pregnant/ trying-to-conceive/tips/success-after-trouble-getting-pregnant/

HealthyWomen Editors. (2014, June 24). *4 Sex tips to help you get pregnant - HealthyWomen*. Healthy Women. https://www.healthywomen.org/your-health/4-sex-tips-help-you-get-pregnant

Hetrick, CNM, P. (2022, October 17). *10 Common pregnancy myths*. University Hospitals. https://www.uhhospitals.org/blog/articles/2022/10/10-common-pregnancy-myths

Ho, MD, J. (2023). *In vitro fertilization overview*. Up To Date. https://www.uptodate.com/contents/in-vitro-fertilization-ivf-beyond-the-basics

I Changed My Narrative From "I Can't Get Pregnant" to "I Can't Wait to Get Pregnant." (2020). Clearblue. https://www.clearblue.com/conceiving hood/stories/saira

Kaufman, C. (2018). *Foods that can affect fertility*. Eatright.org. https://www.eatright.org/health/pregnancy/fertility-and-reproduction/fertility-foods

Kirkwin-Jones, E. (2023, June 16). *13 celebrities who have spoken out about fertility struggles*. Mother & Baby. https://www.motherandbaby.com/getting-pregnant/fertility/celebrities-who-struggled-with-infertility/

Kutteh, W. H., Brezina, P. R., Ke, R. W., & Bailey, A. P. (n.d.). *Infertility myths vs. facts «fertility associates of Memphis*. Fertility Memphis. https://www.fertilitymemphis.com/infertility-myths-2/

Marrocco, J., & McEwen, B. (2016). Sex in the brain: hormones and sex differences. *Sex Differences, 18*(4), 373–383. https://doi.org/10.31887/dcns.2016.18.4/jmarrocco

Mauer, E. D. (2020, March 18). *11 ways to de-stress while you're trying to conceive*. theBump. https://www.thebump.com/a/11-ways-to-de-stress-while-you-re-trying-to-conceive?vers=0

Mayo Clinic Staff. (2021, December 3). *Symptoms of pregnancy: What happens first*. Mayo Clinic. https://www.mayoclinic.org/healthy-life style/getting-pregnant/in-depth/symptoms-of-pregnancy/art-20043853

Mayo Clinic. (2018). *Female infertility - Symptoms and causes*. Mayo

REFERENCES | 191

Clinic. https://www.mayoclinic.org/diseases-conditions/female-infertility/symptoms-causes/syc-20354308

Mayo Clinic. (2019). *Intrauterine insemination (IUI) - Mayo Clinic*. Mayo Clinic. https://www.mayoclinic.org/tests-procedures/intrauterine-insemination/about/pac-20384722

Mayo Clinic. (2021, September 1). *Infertility - Diagnosis and treatment - Mayo Clinic*. Mayo Clinic. https://www.mayoclinic.org/diseases-conditions/infertility/diagnosis-treatment/drc-20354322

Menstrual Cycle (2012). Better Health Channel. https://www.betterhealth.vic.gov.au/health/conditionsandtreatments/menstrual-cycle

Methods for tracking your fertility and ovulation. (2020, September 27). Walnut Hill. https://walnuthillobgyn.com/blog/methods-for-tracking-your-fertility-and-ovulation/

Miracle baby born after difficult pregnancy. (n.d.). Sutter Health https://www.sutterhealth.org/patient-stories/the-molina-family-pregnancy-ob-care

Miscarriage. (2023). March of Dimes. https://www.marchofdimes.org/find-support/topics/miscarriage-loss-grief/miscarriage

Multiple miscarriages. (2023). BostonIVF. https://www.bostonivf.com/our-practice/patient-success-stories/multiple-miscarriages/

9 inspiring infertility stories of hope and determination. (2021). Fertility-Dost. https://www.fertilitydost.com/articles/article-details/9-inspiring-infertility-stories-of-hope-and-determination

Paciuc, MD, J. (n.d.). *8 lifestyle changes that can enhance your fertility: John Paciuc, MD: OBGYN*. John Pacicu, MD. https://www.johnpaciucmd.com/blog/8-lifestyle-changes-that-can-enhance-your-fertility

Pike, A. (2022, June 17). *What is the fertility diet?* Food Insight. https://foodinsight.org/what-is-the-fertility-diet/

Pregnancy - signs and symptoms. (2022, April 16). Better Health Channel. https://www.betterhealth.vic.gov.au/health/HealthyLiving/pregnancy-signs-and-symptoms

Pregnancy after miscarriage: All your questions answered. (n.d.). Flo.health. https://flo.health/pregnancy/pregnancy-health/pregnancy-loss/pregnancy-after-miscarriage

Robinson, K. M. (2022, July 23). *Your best days for making a baby*.

WebMD. https://www.webmd.com/baby/features/best-days-making-baby

Skiadas, MD, C. C. (2023). *Fertility and your weight: How they're connected*. Lancaster General Health. https://www.lancastergeneralhealth.org/health-hub-home/2022/october/fertility-and-your-weight-how-theyre-connected

Tabackman, L. (2021, October 21). *Your first prenatal visit*. Healthline. https://www.healthline.com/health/pregnancy/evaluation-physician#end-of-visit

Tan, D. P. (2021, December 7). *10 ways to support your wife through the fertility treatment process - Dr Pamela Tan*. Dr Pamela Tan Medical Clinic. https://drpamelatan.com/fertility-treatment-process/

Tan, Q., & Cai, X. (n.d.). *Fertility success stories*. Art of Wellness. https://myartofwellness.com/fertility-success-stories/

Weiss, J. (2023, July 11). *Hugh Jackman's 2 kids: Everything to know*. People. https://people.com/parents/all-about-hugh-jackman-kids/

What are the key fertility hormones and what role do they play? (2020, February 17). Forth. https://www.forthwithlife.co.uk/blog/what-are-the-key-fertility-hormones-and-what-role-do-they-play/

Young, J. (n.d.). *Fertility diet success stories | Julia Young nutrition*. Julia Young Nutrition. https://www.juliayoungnutrition.com/fertility-diet-success-stories

Your feelings and emotions after miscarriage. (2019, December 17). Tommy's. https://www.tommys.org/baby-loss-support/miscarriage-information-and-support/support-after-miscarriage/your-feelings-and-emotions-after-miscarriage

Made in the USA
Monee, IL
11 January 2024